Ideologies of Breast Cancer

Feminist Perspectives

Edited by

Laura K. Potts
Senior Tutor in Women's Studies
University College of Ripon and York St John
York

First published in Great Britain 2000 by
MACMILLAN PRESS LTD
Houndmills, Basingstoke, Hampshire RG21 6XS and London
Companies and representatives throughout the world

A catalogue record for this book is available from the British Library.

ISBN 0–333–75419–0 hardcover
ISBN 0–333–75420– 4 paperback

First published in the United States of America 2000 by
ST. MARTIN'S PRESS, INC.,
Scholarly and Reference Division,
175 Fifth Avenue, New York, N.Y. 10010

ISBN 0–312–22851–1

Library of Congress Cataloging-in-Publication Data
Ideologies of breast cancer : feminist perspectives / edited by Laura
K. Potts.
p. cm.
Includes bibliographical references and index.
ISBN 0–312–22851–1 (cloth)
1. Breast—Cancer. 2. Breast—Cancer—Social aspects.
3. Feminism. 4. Women—Medical care. I. Potts, Laura.
RC280.B8I34 1999
616.99'449—dc21   99–37438
                                                                CIP

This book is printed on paper suitable for recycling and made from fully managed and sustained
forest sources.

10   9   8   7   6   5   4   3   2   1
09 08 07 06 05 04 03 02 01 00

Printed and bound in Great Britain by
Antony Rowe Ltd, Chippenham, Wiltshire

22 April 1992

*Everything takes longer
than you think it should
or thought it would.
Except your life.*

Merijane Block

Contents

Preface   ix

Acknowledgements   xi

Notes on the Contributors   xii

Introduction: Why Ideologies of Breast Cancer? Why Feminist
Perspectives?
Laura K. Potts   1

PART I Meanings of Breast Cancer

1. Problematizing Biomedicine: Women's Constructions of
   Breast Cancer Knowledge
   Jennifer Fosket   15

2. Sexualized Illness: the Newsworthy Body in Media
   Representations of Breast Cancer
   Cherise Saywell, with Lesley Henderson and Liza Beattie   37

3. Racing for the Cure, Walking Women and Toxic Touring:
   Mapping Cultures of Action within the Bay Area Terrain
   of Breast Cancer
   Maren Klawiter   63

4. Publishing the Personal: Autobiographical Narratives of
   Breast Cancer and the Self
   Laura K. Potts   98

PART II Discourses of Risk and Breast Cancer

5. Controversies in Breast Cancer Prevention: the Discourse
   of Risk
   Christy Simpson   131

6. Reconstructing the Body or Reconstructing the Woman?
   Problems of Prophylactic Mastectomy for Hereditary Breast
   Cancer Risk
   Nina Hallowell   153

7. Assessing Breast Cancer: Risk, Science and Environmental
    Activism in an 'At Risk' Community
    Jennifer Fishman   181

Index   205

Preface

This book, in the form in which you hold it, is the realization of an idea that came to me one hot afternoon in Kingston, Ontario, at the First Worldwide Conference on Breast Cancer in July 1997. Its previous incarnation as a co-authored text had been abandoned just a few months earlier, but the stimulus of hearing so many committed and lively women express their ideas about breast cancer (as well as the inspirational accounts of activism and research, support and self-help), made a reconfiguring of the original concept seem possible. And so I enthusiastically approached some of the women whose papers I had particularly found interesting, for the ways in which they touched on but moved beyond some of the original shaping ideas for the book, and began to consider how the book project might be reborn.

Working with other people's ideas in addition to my own has certainly been a much more enjoyable and exciting project than struggling alone with the limitations of my intellectual parameters and fluctuating levels of enthusiasm – like being involved in a seminar where both speaking and listening begin to inform new ways of understanding and to generate different visions. Thus I trust that the book is more than the sum of its parts; that the connections and inter-relationships are visible and provocative; that each chapter presents a particular perspective that sheds light on the others, even as it retains its integrity as a discrete and well-constructed piece of analysis in its own right.

Of course, this privileged view of the whole has, until now, until publication, been mine alone, and the 'seminar' effect has, paradoxically, been my singular experience. Writing about breast cancer from within any discipline, and from whatever discursive position, is an uncomfortable and at times distressing activity. None of us who has contributed chapters here has breast cancer; but we all know women who have, and have worked closely with women who have. And, inevitably, while the incidence of the disease continues to rise in those countries from which we write (UK, USA, Canada), and scant attention is paid to primary prevention, we are likely to know more and more women with breast cancer, and so is the reader. Given the broad but overarching feminist perspectives from which the book comes, the contributors' position may be seen as one of standing alongside those women. For the time being we may think, 'There but for the grace . . .'.

The closeness to other women's stories each contributor has heard or read brings particular strains to the process of writing, and at times the isolation that is of that process has made the work particularly difficult. This observation is in no way intended to diminish or to detract from the far more acute and immediate distress and isolation of the women whose breast cancer we account for here. I want rather to acknowledge the efforts of the contributors to this book, knowing from my own experience during its production, and from the e-mail and telephone conversations with the others, that it has been unusually hard to stay with the work to this point of publication. The intention was to generate greater understanding of breast cancer, in all but clinical terms; to consider the meanings and significances it has in contemporary, northern over-developed societies. For their part in ensuring that illumination is vivid, compelling and innovative, I thank all the contributors profoundly.

Acknowledgements

I would like to thank those people who gave me the support to realize the aim of producing this book: most of all, my pal Pat Spallone, who has been involved from the very beginning – always enthusiastic, always a critical visionary, who listened to vague ideas and helped make them material, and offered detailed commentary on early drafts of my own chapter. She made this project possible at the crucial level of belief and encouragement, along with Mary Eagleton, Liz Maynard, Judy Giles and Trev Broughton, from Women's Studies in York; several other colleagues and friends made it possible by their practical support, and I particularly thank Chris Clay and Greg Lodge at UCRYSJ for negotiating my sabbatical leave at a difficult time for them. Jane Tyler's generosity with her time and technological expertise, as well as with the long-term loan of her neat portable computer, made the whole project less awesome and helped me get there in the end.

In sisterhood,
Laura Potts, York

Notes on the Contributors

Liza Beattie is a researcher at the Media Research Unit, University of Glasgow. Key research areas include the production, content and reception of media messages in relation to racism, migration and the developing world. She is currently researching a PhD on this theme with the University of Bradford.

Jennifer Fishman is a doctoral student in sociology in the Department of Social and Behavioral Sciences at the University of California, San Francisco. Her research interests include: the sociology of the environment, medical, and technological risks and uncertainties; feminist theories; science and technology studies; and the sociology of biomedical and scientific knowledge.

Jennifer Fosket is a doctoral student in sociology at the University of California, San Francisco, where she has worked as a breast cancer researcher on several social science studies. Her dissertation research focuses on the sociology of breast cancer research, science and prevention. She is also actively engaged in numerous activities within the larger breast cancer community.

Nina Hallowell is a Senior Research Associate in the Centre for Family Research at Cambridge University, England. She has qualifications in psychology and general linguistics. Her research interests include: women's health, the psychosocial implications of new genetic technologies, and the sociology of risk and the body. She is currently working on a research project which looks at the information needs of women who are making decisions about preventative surgery because they have a family history of ovarian cancer.

Lesley Henderson is a Research Fellow at the Mass Media Research Unit, University of Glasgow. She is currently researching the influence of media on women's infant feeding choices. She has written previously on media representations of health/illness.

Maren Klawiter is a PhD candidate in the Department of Sociology, University of California, Berkeley. Her dissertation, 'Reshaping the

Contours of Breast Cancer: From Private Stigma to Cultures of Action' is based upon more than three years of ethnographic research within the San Francisco Bay Area field of activism, and historical research on changes in the screening, surveillance and medical treatment of asymptomatic populations, women diagnosed with ambiguous conditions, and women diagnosed with breast cancer. In the autumn of 1999 she begins a two-year postdoctoral position as a Robert Wood Johnson Scholar in Health Policy Research at the University of Michigan, Ann Arbor, where she will be examining the shift from treating disease to treating the condition of being 'at risk' for breast cancer, focusing on the production of 'risky subjects' and the deployment of new 'risk-reduction' biotechnologies.

Laura K. Potts is Senior Tutor for Women's Studies in the Faculty of Social, Environmental, Health and Life Sciences at the University College of Ripon and York St John, in York, UK. Her initial academic study was in literature and philosophy, with further work in health education. She has taught widely in adult, further and higher education for many years while also maintaining an involvement in feminist activism and women's health (currently as a member of 'free radicals', campaigning on breast cancer and the environment), and organic food growing. Her other research interests include women's friendship, auto/biography, and the politics and sociology of food. Her poetry has been published in various anthologies.

Cherise Saywell is a researcher at the Glasgow Media Research Unit. She completed a master's degree in communications and cultural studies at the University of Queensland in Brisbane, Australia. Her main research interests involve media representations of women's issues, focusing primarily on sexuality and health-related topics. She has previously worked in Australia on projects about HIV and AIDS as well as breast cancer, and is currently working on an NHS Executive-funded project about public and professional understandings of breast cancer.

Christy Simpson is a PhD candidate in philosophy at Dalhousie University, Nova Scotia, Canada. She has a long-standing interest in cancer, starting first from a biological/scientific research perspective that has now changed to a bioethics/feminist perspective. Her master's dissertation focused on risk assessment in breast cancer. Presentations related to this work have been made at various conferences including the First World Conference on Breast Cancer. Having been raised on a dairy farm in Ontario, Canada, she is a practical person concerned with the application of philosophy to concrete situations, as in her work in clinical oncology at local hospitals. Her studies have been supported by an Ontario Graduate Scholarship, an Izaak Walton Killam Memorial Scholarship, and a Social Science and Humanities Research Council Doctoral Fellowship.

Introduction: Why Ideologies of Breast Cancer? Why Feminist Perspectives?

Laura K. Potts

The prime concern in this collection of critical essays is to reveal the meanings that breast cancer has in contemporary society, not just for those women immediately affected by it or for those involved in working with those who are, but more broadly, as a common and present reality in all our lives. Notable work has been done by Sontag (1989) and by Stacey (1997) in illuminating the meanings cancer has in the contemporary northern/western (over-)developed world: the fear of growth, the inferences of invasion and of uncontrollability, the sense of monstrosity and the metaphors of war that are invoked. The justification for looking more specifically at breast cancer is primarily one of the relevance granted by the prevalence of the disease in those societies, by the fact that it will directly touch the lives of one in eleven women in the UK, and as many as one in eight in some areas of the United States, at some point, and inevitably, indirectly, many more, as friends, partners, colleagues, sisters, mothers, daughters ... There are frequent reminders of this threat, perpetuated through the popular media as well as through personal contacts, so that the idea of breast cancer has become a lived reality for most post-pubertal women. The message is now annually reinforced to 'well women' in Britain and North America by the designation of October as Breast Cancer Awareness Month – a notion dreamed up by Imperial Chemical Industries (ICI) and now largely managed and controlled by Zeneca, a multinational chemical/pharmaceuticals corporation.[1]

Meaning can be revealed through examination of the particular beliefs, values, socio-cultural practices and the dominant tropes pertaining to a topic, and it is in relation to this process of examination that an understanding of inherent ideologies is of critical

1

importance. For, as Althusser (quoted in Fuss 1989: 114) says, 'When we speak of ideology we should know that ideology slides into all human activity, that it is identical with the "lived" experience of human existence itself ... This "lived" experience is not a given, given by a pure "reality", but the spontaneous "lived experience" of ideology in its particular relationship to the real'. It is the relationship between ideology and the real that was of particular interest to me in collecting the essays for this book, for it is in the deconstruction of that relationship, and the insights acquired through that process, that a clearer understanding of the role of breast cancer in all our lives becomes apparent. I feel no need to claim any particular therapeutic or applied health benefit from that understanding, though those certainly may also be outcomes of that work, believing rather that intellectual insights, new perspectives and the creation of new knowledges do in and of themselves shift the ideological terrain we inhabit, and thus the 'lived reality' we experience.

While Althusser's project involved a dissolving of the subject, the intention here is rather to assert the very presence of the subjects, of the women who live with the reality of breast cancer as threat or actuality. Such an emphasis is central to feminist thinking and practice, an assertion against the invisibility and silence which cloak so many women's lives. By emphasizing 'feminist perspectives', that particular validation of women's experiences is signalled; the contributions here illuminate the variety of stories and of socially constructed meanings which breast cancer has, but each chapter's analysis is a location in which women's lives are made visible and their voices heard. This is the specific context for my own chapter, which is concerned with the stories women tell to make sense of their experiences of breast cancer, and with the narrative construction of personal and collective meaning. All the contributions in the book are methodologically constructed, whatever their discretely diverse academic approaches, to ensure that a crucial starting point for research and enquiry is the lived experience of women themselves; it is through these means that new knowledge and a new sense of what breast cancer signifies can be seen to emerge. The chapters thus manifest what Dorothy Smith has described as 'the project of a sociology for women; that is, a sociology which does not transform those it studies into objects but preserves in its analytic procedures the presence of the subject as actor and experiencer' (Smith 1988). This is the ideological and feminist take on breast cancer which the book aims to provide, what Harding (quoted by Rose 1994: 84) suggests is so radical in Smith's approach to the social sciences: '[a] fusing [of] hitherto "incompatible tendencies towards interpretation, explanation and critical theory"'.

The contributions to this book are not, however, located within any one intellectual discipline; they draw on a wide range of discursive methods and practices. A broadly sociological bias may be discerned, but this, I believe, reflects a shared belief among the authors that 'health matters … are profoundly social in cause and consequence' (Petersen and Waddell 1998: vii), rather than any academic conviction of the primacy of the discipline. So the chapters draw on feminist theory and philosophy, on cultural and media studies, on bioethics, on literary criticism, on psychology and sociology, to inform an analysis of the meanings of breast cancer and of the ideologies that inhere in it. 'Evidence' is drawn from interviews with women who have breast cancer, who are 'at risk' of breast cancer and from a general population; from popular media sources; from participation in activism around breast cancer; from the natural and empirical sciences; from published narratives of having the disease, and, of course, from a correspondingly wide-ranging literature review of other people's work related to these areas. This broad and eclectic approach reflects, to use a cancer metaphor, the widespread and differentiated spread of thinking about breast cancer into all the areas of our lives. This is not a subject, not a story, that can be kept bounded, contained within either the clinical or the medico-psychological discourses which still dominate much else that is written on the subject. By applying a range of critical methods, and by their juxtaposition within one volume, and by highlighting women's standpoints in relation to the issues raised, our understanding of how breast cancer is enacted and encoded is revealed more clearly. Therein lies the strength and the impact of bringing women's voices together from diverse fields of activity and work; it is also, I believe, the strength of the kind of inter- and multidisciplinary analysis which characterizes Women's Studies.

The literature on breast cancer is extensive; even excluding the vast amount of medical and medico-psychological research published all over the world, the range of information and commentary is very considerable. The last decade of English language publishing has certainly seen something of a welcome shift towards the inclusion of perspectives expressed by women with breast cancer themselves, but the emphases still tend to be of expert opinion bestowed upon the 'ill-informed', or of insider talk from one member of the breast cancer cognoscenti to another. The intention here is rather to consider the ideological discourses in which breast cancer is variously constructed and, in particular, to examine the ways in which feminist perspectives are able 'both to appropriate and make over powerful tools hitherto marked for the discourse of mastery' (Rose 1994: 74). In this context, Dorothy Smith's concept of the use of the term 'ideology' may help to focus the reader's mind on particular issues of concern in the book as a whole. She writes:

> I am not using the term to refer to political beliefs ... nor ... to draw the boundaries between an impartial and disinterested social science and 'ideology' as an interested and partial perspective ... I am concerned, rather, with ideology as those ideas and images through which the class that rules society ... orders, organizes, and sanctions the social relations that sustain its domination ... Thus, the concept of ideology ... directs us to look for and at the actual practical organization of the production of images, ideas, symbols, concepts, vocabularies, as means for us to think about our world. (Smith 1988: 54)

The individual chapters will reveal to the reader the diverse emphases of that range of discourses within particular social environments, and how they inform the particular life experiences of women.

Breast cancer has been claimed as a feminist issue in a variety of ways. Wilkinson and Kitzinger quote Nancy Datan, a feminist psychologist who died of breast cancer, thus: 'It is a central tenet of feminism that women's invisible and private wounds often reflect social and political injustices. It is a commitment central to feminism to share burdens. And it is an axiom of feminism that the personal is political' (Wilkinson and Kitzinger 1994: 124). Earlier critiques of breast cancer treatment and diagnosis (such as Choice and Control in Breast Disease, in *Our Bodies Ourselves,* eds. Phillips and Rakusen, 1988) tended to address these three defining pointers by asserting the need for improved access to, and sharing of, information and for the right to greater choice and control by women in relation to a disease largely managed by medical men given power by virtue of their profession as well as their gender. Pragmatically, much has changed since those times: the incorporation into mainstream healthcare delivery of a feminist rhetoric, with its emphasis on empowerment through the sharing of experience, the greater availability of accessible information, and on choice of care and treatment, is some kind of a success story for the Women's Health Movement of the 1980s. Self-help and support groups and information giving are now generally, if not wholeheartedly and universally, acknowledged by the mainstream healthcare providers to be 'a good thing', at least as long as they do not directly challenge the clinical hegemony of medical staff.[2]

The increased acceptance of 'alternative' or 'complementary' medicine has followed a similar trajectory, albeit that the 'soft' end of that spectrum of therapies is the most readily incorporated, with some UK breast care nurses recommending aromatherapy, while acupuncture and nutritional therapy are more likely still to be perceived as outside medical norms. Patients' views are now, ostensibly, sought, and information needs are, ostensibly, recognized too, as the range of published papers on the topic testifies. (A meta-analysis of such work is currently being researched at the NHS Centre for Review and Dissemination at the University of York, England.) Such examples of 'progress', of positive change in relation to the perception and treatment of breast cancer, tend to be regarded as evidence of a more woman- or patient-centred model, in which choice and control have been significantly devolved to her and away from the medical profession. Other interpretations may also, however, be suggested, in which such changes may be regarded, if not with a jaundiced eye, then at least with a more critical and sharper vision which includes a closer look at the 'relations of ruling', to use Smith's (1988) term, and how they maintain authority over the ways in which we think about breast cancer.

In many respects, while the predominant ideologies of breast cancer are configured within a modernist paradigm of progress and improvement, they are rendered problematic by the adoption of alternative standpoints, as the contributions here make clear. But perhaps the most telling of arguments questioning the norm of optimistic progress for women in relation to breast cancer, and the assertion that choice and control are enhanced, is articulated by environmental campaigners who claim that our risk of developing the disease is significantly raised by contaminants in our everyday lives over which we have no control whatsoever (see, for example, Read 1995; and Women's Environmental Network 1998). There has, significantly, been little discernible change in terms of the acceptability of a discourse which attends to the primary prevention of the disease, despite its rising incidence in most countries. The main emphases in almost all references to breast cancer are still on treatment, reconstruction and genetic factors, as Saywell's research shows. This is not least because the primary prevention of breast cancer would demand the validation of arguments that challenge the 'cancer industry' (a term adopted by

activists in the Bay Area of California, who mark breast cancer awareness month with a 'Toxic Tour' of the cancer industries implicated in
causing breast cancer, as Klawiter's chapter describes), and assert the
political rights of women not just to information, which, after all, is
still largely mediated and controlled through the establishment, but
to protection from the environmental carcinogens that contribute to
the aetiology of the disease. Rachel Carson articulated these arguments as long ago as 1962 (Carson 1991), and other environmental
campaigners continue to emphasize similar points (Steingraber 1998;
Read 1995; Epstein et al. 1997). Fishman's chapter vividly reveals how
those discourses are silenced by researchers – both natural and social
scientists – working ostensibly for the community living in a particularly contaminated part of the San Francisco Bay Area, where the
incidence of breast cancer is the highest in the world.

The widespread adoption of mass screening programmes, following
the trials in Sweden in the 1980s (see, for instance, Shapiro 1982;
Verbeek 1984; Tabar 1985; Forrest 1986) has effectively persuaded
most women of the need for technological surveillance of their breasts
at medically determined intervals, in the name of their health,
empowerment and autonomy. This is reinforced in the 1990s by
injunctions to women to be 'breast aware', to attend screening when
offered, and to practise regular breast self-examination. These developments, too, may be understood within a modernist paradigm or
challenged from a more critical standpoint. The services are designed
to encourage women to attend, and to pay attention, often by the
design of more female-friendly environments, be they clinics with
flowery wallpaper or leaflets trying hard to express their message in
what is perceived to be the vernacular of a particular target group.
Compliance is still, however, the main aim of such programmes, with
high take-up rates set because the benefits of mammography are reck-
oned on a population basis, and thus are only realizable if a maximum
percentage of that population attends. The message is that early breast
cancer can be treated successfully, and that all women should avail
themselves of the opportunities offered by screening to ensure that
any cancer is detected early, whether by mammography for older
women, or by self-examination. This is in fact a distortion of a more
complex reality, a 'telescop[ing] ... of subtle truths into a saleable
mantra' (Stabiner 1997: 168). As Susan Love explains:

'Mammograms can see eighty-five percent of breast cancers' ...
They may already be the size of a grapefruit, but we can see them.

Then we say, 'Mammograms can find cancer early,' which is also true. They can't always, but sometimes they can. Then we say, 'Early cancer is ninety-five percent curable.' Which is true – at least according to the admittedly untrustworthy five-year survival marker. 'So when you say those three sentences fast, one after another, you come away thinking, 'Mammograms can find eighty-five percent of cancers when they're ninety-five percent curable.' Which is not true at all. (*ibid.*)

So the increased technologically and empirically-driven surveillance of health and potential disease states demands that women take on the scientific discourse of breast cancer and match the supposed clinical vigilance with a personal attentiveness to changes in their breasts, which they are then supposed to refer to the health and illness authorities. This construction corresponds to the postmodern movement of medicine from a unitary location within the clinic into a variety of other micro-locations in society, which yet retain the discursive identity of their origins. But such a domestication of health practices further requires women to negotiate the resulting range of complex different contextual interpretations of their bodies, the risk of breast cancer and the management of disease. As Fosket's chapter demonstrates, this necessarily demands negotiation and interaction with different knowledge sets, from the biomedical/empirical/positivist to the intuitive/personal/particular, and an engagement with a complicated appraisal of the reliability of those different accounts. Her chapter provides crucial critical insights into the question of just how empowering those multiple positions really are, and into the implicit tension that characterizes the various meanings and significances which the disease thus acquires. Simpson similarly shows how women are required to undertake risk assessment of their own likelihood of developing breast cancer, by recourse to a weighing up of information which is contradictory and difficult to understand.

'Information is power' was an implicit slogan of the 1980s Women's Health Movement, with an allied assumption being that empowered women would have more control over their lives and bodies. The new emphasis on genetic and heritable determinants of breast cancer, since the discovery of the marker genes BRCA1 and BRCA2 in 1994, provides, however, a clear illustration of the more problematic social context of having information about one's own body. As Hallowell's chapter shows, women who are found to have a genetic mutation and therefore are deemed to be at 'high risk' of developing breast cancer, face a range of 'choices' which are not necessarily empowering at all and confer little real personal autonomy. Rather, this new information, and the discourse in which it is constructed, demand of these women a confrontation with their own 'dangerous' bodies and potentially compromised sense of femininity, while recourse to clinical intervention is seen as the sole means of resolving those conflicts. The discourse of risk in relation to breast cancer is not, however, entirely amenable to the same analysis as that posited in other recent critiques of health risk discourse (Lupton 1995; Bunton 1992; Lupton and Petersen 1996). While the broader dominant rhetoric of breast cancer management may now be established as one of women having choice and control, and corresponds to other aspects of postmodern healthcare in so far as risk analysis and management become the responsibility of the actively vigilant consumer, breast cancer risk remains a problem that is only to be addressed by medical intervention. Popular discourse does not yet account breast cancer as a risk that may be avoided by attention to lifestyle, and thus while women are urged to manage risk through techniques of self-surveillance as described above, the governance of that 'high risk population' remains the responsibility of science and technology. Thus the monitoring of the self of which Giddens (1991) writes cannot, in the context of breast cancer, be an individual project, but has to be negotiated through pharmacological or surgical prophylaxis, as Simpson's and Hallowell's chapters respectively consider.

One further ideological discourse importantly informs the way in which the disease is understood and the meanings it has. As Saywell's chapter clearly demonstrates, constructions of embodied femininity impact both individually and collectively on women and significantly shape the cultural valorization of reconstruction, or the re-normalization of the visible female body. Some feminist critiques of breast cancer treatment used to emphasize the neglect by surgeons of women's fear of the mutilating effects of surgery, and of mastectomy in particular (Rosser 1991; Morris 1983). Those concerns have been addressed during the last decade, but appropriated by the surgeons themselves, within a medical discourse aligned with their colleagues from psycho-oncology and entirely circumscribed by the normative assumptions of breast shape, size and significance (see Baum 1988; Fallowfield 1991). The challenge to this dominant discourse of the desirability of retaining a woman's 'wholeness' and 'femininity' by conservative surgery and the construction of prosthetic breasts, which was articulated by Lorde (1980) nearly twenty years ago, seems only to have been taken up within particular cultural milieux: by lesbian women in their own communities; by feminists in 'safe' environments; or by those who already position themselves outside a cultural norm, like Kathy Acker. Images of ideal femininity may have changed in the two decades to which I am referring here, but they remain unexceptionally informed by an ideal of two-breasted symmetry.

This, then, is an introductory overview of the main ideological discourses examined in the book. It will, I hope, serve to whet the reader's appetite – without spoiling it by offering too much of a taster of what the contributors themselves have to say. The purpose here has rather been to set a general scene, historically and politically, so that the meanings and emphases given by the individual chapters are usefully contextualized for the reader, and a rationale for the particular titular focus of the book established as a cohesive focus.

Notes

1 As well as being the fourth largest producer of pesticides in the US – and there is considerable evidence of the contribution of organochlorine pesticide use to breast cancer (Women's Environmental Network 1998) – Zeneca manufacture the most widely prescribed drug for breast cancer, tamoxifen, used both in treatment and as prophylaxis in 'high-risk' women; the corporation also owns a management company which runs a chain of cancer care centres in the US (Brady 1997).

2 Klawiter offers a detailed critical analysis of these shifts in her paper *Breast Cancer in Two Regimes;* using a case study of Clara Larson, who has had breast cancer twice, in 1979 and in 1997, she shows how the socio-medical environment in which Clara experiences the disease has shifted from 'the breast cancer regime of physician sovereignty' to 'the breast health regime of biosociety'. While her observational analysis is culturally situated within the specific context of the Bay Area of California, the trajectory of change she identifies is more generally applicable; in the new regime, she states 'there arose new flows of information, new social networks, and new forms of connection and community'. In part this can be explained as a movement away from the clinic and a unified clinical gaze, towards an environment of health and illness which subjects a population to a multiple gaze from an expanded treatment team and from a culture of self-surveillance, where health is constantly emphasized and highlighted. This analysis is valid for any of the social cultures considered in the book, and can be configured alongside other postmodern trends defining new social configurations. But there are more precisely located observations in Klawiter's work, which offer a careful situational positioning of the changing terrain of the ideological construction of breast cancer. She shows clearly how the women with breast cancer whom she has studied over a period of several years are no longer so much required to 'navigate their cancer diagnoses and treatments in discursive silence, social isolation,

medical ignorance, and cultural invisibility', and locates this changed land-scape in its particularity. Given those new means of networking and sharing information, the defining characteristics of a specific social, temporal and geographical trend become singularly focused, and it is certainly possible now to identify an international breast cancer movement which, while retaining some features of local specificity, is also able to merge and incorporate ideas and strategies from other locations.

References

Baum, M. *Breast Cancer: The Facts,* 2nd edition (Oxford: Oxford University Press 1988).

Brady, J. 'Public Relations and Cancer', in Women's Cancer Resource Center's *Center News* (Berkeley: WCRC 1997).

Bunton, R. 'More than a wooly jumper: health promotion as social regulation', *Critical Public Health,* vol. 3, no. 2 (1992) pp. 4–11.

Carson, R. *Silent Spring* (Harmondsworth: Penguin 1991; first published 1962).

Epstein, S. et al. *The Breast Cancer Prevention Program* (London: Macmillan 1997).

Fallowfield, L. with A. Clark. *Breast Cancer* (London: Tavistock/Routledge 1991).

Forrest, P. et al. *Breast Cancer Screening: Report to the Health Ministers of Engalnd, Wales, Scotland and Northern Ireland* (London: HMSO 1986).

Fuss, D. *Essentially Speaking: Feminism, Nature and Difference* (London: Routledge 1989).

Giddens, A. *Modernity and Self-Identity: Self and Society in the Late Modern Age* (Cambridge: Polity Press 1991).

Klawiter, M. 'Breast Cancer in Two Regimes', Introduction to forthcoming doctoral thesis at University of California, Berkeley.

Lorde, A. *The Cancer Journals* (San Francisco: Spinsters Ink 1980).

Lupton, D. and A. Petersen. *The New Public Health: Health and Self in the Age of Risk* (Sydney: Allan and Unwin 1996)

Lupton, D. *The Imperative of Health: Public Health and the Regulated Body* (London: Sage 1995).

Morris, T. 'Psycho-social Aspects of Breast Cancer: A Review', *European Journal of Cancer and Critical Oncology* 19(12) (1983) pp.1725–35.

Petersen, A. and C. Waddell. *Health Matters, A Sociology of Illness, Prevention and Care* (Buckingham: Open University Press 1998).

Phillips, A. and J. Rakusen, eds., *The New Our Bodies Ourselves* (Harmondsworth: Penguin 1989).

Read, C. *Preventing Breast Cancer, the Study of an Epidemic* (London: Pandora 1995).

Rose, H. *Love, Power and Knowledge: Towards a Feminist Transformation of the Sciences* (Cambridge: Polity Press 1994).

Rosser, J.E. 'The Interpretation of Women's Experience: A Critical Appraisal of the Literature on Breast Cancer', *Social Science and Medicine,* 15E (1991) pp. 257–65.

Shapiro, S 'Ten to Fourteen Year Effect of Screening on Breast Cancer Mortality'. *Journal of the National Cancer Institute,* vol. 62, no. 2 (1982).

Smith, D. *The Everyday World as Problematic: A Feminist Sociology* (Milton Keynes: Open University Press 1988).

Sontag, S. *Illness as Metaphor* (Harmondsworth: Penguin 1977).

Stabiner, K. *To Dance with the Devil: The New War on Breast Cancer, Politics, Power, People* (New York: Bantam Doubleday Dell 1997).

Stacey, J. *Teratologies, a Cultural Study of Cancer* (London: Routledge 1997).

Steingraber, S. *Living Downstream: An Ecologist Looks at Cancer and the Environment* (London: Little, Brown and Co. 1998).

Tabar, L. et al. 'Reduction in Mortality from Breast Cancer after Mass Screening with Mammography'. *The Lancet* (13 April 1985) pp. 829–32.

Verbeek, A.L. et al. 'Reduction of Breast Cancer Mortality through Mass Screening with Modern Mammographs', *The Lancet*, vol. i, (1984) pp. 1222–6.

Wilkinson, S. and C. Kitzinger. 'Towards a Feminist Approach to Breast Cancer', in Wilkinson, S. and C. Kitzinger, eds. *Women and Health, Feminist Perspectives* (London: Taylor and Francis 1994).

Women's Environmental Network. *Putting Breast Cancer on the Map* (London: WEN 1998).

Part I
Meanings of Breast Cancer

1
Problematizing Biomedicine: Women's Constructions of Breast Cancer Knowledge

Jennifer Fosket

In the United States, breast cancer is a disease about which there exist multiple, often conflictual and complex knowledges. The multiplicity of knowledges about breast cancer is interesting and important, not just for the epistemological questions it raises regarding how knowledges come to be constructed, but also for the political questions regarding what is at stake in different knowledge constructions. And a lot is at stake. Breast cancer is a disease that robs 44,000 US women of their lives each year and thus many, many women's lives are at stake in the processes of constructing knowledge about breast cancer. It is a disease for which treatments are brutal, painful and life-altering and thus the lives of the 180,000 women who are diagnosed in the US each year are at stake. There are no known causes of breast cancer, except radiation, and thus, the lives of all women are at stake because with no known causes, there can be no real prevention. With an enormous amount of money spent each year on diagnosis and treatment, breast cancer is also a big industry and big business; for the pharmaceutical and biotechnological companies that produce treatment and diagnostic technologies, there is therefore a lot of money at stake. Tremendous amounts of money are also granted to breast cancer research each year and thus, there is also a lot of money at stake for researchers and funding agencies. Additionally, there are financial implications, reputations, jobs, prestige and collegial networks to be gained by breast cancer researchers from the knowledges that they produce. There is also money for the companies and products that sponsor Breast Cancer Awareness Month and other commercialization-of-breast-cancer projects. Within the breast cancer activist movements, what is at stake is the moral authority to speak for communities of women with breast cancer, in terms both of how, as well as what, knowledges are constructed.

The proliferation of individuals and groups concerned with breast cancer and their diversity of commitments and interests are reflected in the variations on the knowledges produced about breast cancer – how it is framed and what it means. Breast cancer causation, detection strategies and guidelines, treatment options and effectiveness, who is at risk, the meaning of incidence and mortality statistics, and the possibility of a cure are the pre-eminent among these multiple knowledge sites, and where controversies abound. Different knowledges about breast cancer are produced by social movements, by women with breast cancer, by those critical of biomedicine and by biomedicine itself. These controversies abound both 'within' as well as 'outside' the traditional, biomedical realm of knowledge production and problematize the notion of a clear boundary between 'inside' and 'outside' biomedicine, or between 'biomedical' and 'alternative' knowledges.

In this chapter I explore the multiple ways in which women with breast cancer construct knowledge about their disease. Examining women's constructions of breast cancer knowledge reveals the very real consequences of the complexity and uncertainty of knowledges about breast cancer. While in dominant discourse, breast cancer is viewed as a purely biomedically known and knowable disease entity, for women living with breast cancer it is much more than that.[1] By exploring constructions of knowledge of breast cancer as a biomedical concept, I do not intend to reify the idea that breast cancer can best be understood biomedically. Instead, I hope that such an exploration will accomplish just the opposite, highlighting the ways in which even biomedical constructions are profoundly social and emerge out of the complexities of women's experiences and their interactions and positions in society. These biomedically defined arenas of women's experiences of breast cancer are but a few of the multiple arenas in which breast cancer is lived and in which knowledge of breast cancer is constructed. It is here that I focus my attention because the site offers the important potential to explore the convergence of lived experience and biomedical discourse – of biomedical discourse *as* lived experience – and the resulting construction of biomedicine as contestable and uncertain.

To accomplish this, I first explore ways in which women's stories highlight the political and social nature of biomedical knowledge constructions, thereby challenging the popular depiction of biomedical knowledge as purely objective, always certain, asocial and unproblematic. Secondly, I assert that women's constructions of knowledge highlight both the power of the 'clinical gaze' (Foucault 1973) to name and diagnose illness, without excluding embodied and other knowledge sources that the women simultaneously draw on in constructing their own knowledge of breast cancer. Thirdly, I examine ways that these different knowledge constructions about breast cancer are treated unequally: the ways in which women's knowledges are often dismissed in biomedical interactions around breast cancer through the hierarchy of credibility (Becker 1967) that emerges.

I conclude the chapter by arguing that attentiveness to women's experiences with breast cancer challenges current, taken-for-granted assumptions about breast cancer. Here, I explore ways in which knowledge about breast cancer that is constructed by dominant biomedical experts does not rely on lived experiences to construct its truths and can, as a result, contradict lived, emotional and embodied experiences of breast cancer. By focusing on women's own experiences with breast cancer and the knowledges derived from those experiences, I underscore the ways that dominant biomedical knowledge often falls short of articulating the truths that women come to know through their own experiences.

Methods

This chapter draws on data from a qualitative study in which nine women with breast cancer were interviewed and asked about their experiences, ideas and knowledges about breast cancer and how those ideas and thoughts have changed throughout their experiences. The interviews took place in the women's homes and lasted from one to two hours. I audio taped and transcribed each interview. I coded the transcripts according the Grounded Theory Method laid out by Strauss and Corbin (1990), which yielded the categories for analysis. I drew on the categories I was developing in subsequent interviews, as grounded theory emphasizes a dynamic process of data collection occurring simultaneous to analysis. In this way, the project develops according to what is significant in the data. After completing the initial coding and categorizing, I identified key concepts in the data. These key concepts are the basis for this chapter.

The nine women I interviewed were primarily middle-class, with one working class and one upper middle-class woman. Class is particularly difficult to assess for women who are experiencing potentially prolonged illnesses like breast cancer because such experiences are expensive, can mean leaving work and thus drastically shift one's class position in a short period of time. Five of the nine women I interviewed described either a need to leave work or other potential economic hardships, such as lack of full insurance coverage as a result of their illness. In terms of race and ethnicity, the nine women identified as Latina, white, Filipina or bi-racial. The women ranged in age from 31 to 73 with the majority being in their fifties. Three of the women had had recurrences and six of the women were undergoing treatment at the time of our interview.

Biomedical Knowledges

Within the sociology of knowledge, theorists have long argued that knowledge is constructed within specific situated, historical contexts (e.g. Mannheim 1952). Historically, however, scientific knowledge has been seen as separate, asocial, universal and consequently not subjected to the same theoretical or historical deconstruction and unmasking of interests as other types of knowledge (Ward 1996; Wright and Treacher 1982). Biomedical knowledge both derives from and aligns with science in order to bolster its legitimacy and has thus traditionally shared this exempt status (Estes and Binney 1989; Wright and Treacher 1982). Medical knowledge has been seen as the benevolent application of the objective knowledge derived through scientific methods. Further, the object towards which medical knowledge is utilized – disease – was assumed to be a 'natural' phenomenon, existing outside of and prior to its recognition by medical knowledge (Wright and Treacher, 1982). It is only more recently that theorists have begun to cast a critical gaze towards biomedical and technoscientific knowledge production and dissemination (Lock and Kaufert 1998; Lock and Gordon 1988; Wright and Treacher 1982; Estes and Binney, 1989).

The traditional conflation of biomedical knowledge with truth and objectivity means that the profoundly social and constructed nature of such knowledge is often overlooked, ignored or denied. Discursively, biomedical knowledge is legitimated as adhering to objective standards of truth and method that are seen as removed from culture. Such knowledge is claimed to be beyond culture – universal. On the other hand, knowledge that is not legitimated is often claimed to be local, indigenous or culturally specific, possibly approved in its local context, but dismissed as applicable or valid beyond that specific culture. Legitimate knowledges make a claim to universality in an attempt to decontextualize and erase the cultural elements of its production. Culture is viewed as something that can be transcended in the interest of truth. Here, I argue that in practice, cultural, embodied and experiential knowledges are always drawn upon in the construction of biomedical knowledge just as in other knowledges, even when at the same time such 'illegitimate' sources of knowledges are dismissed as unreliable or illegitimate ways of constructing biomedical knowledge. By focusing on women's constructions of biomedical knowledge, the cultured and social contexts of biomedical knowledge production are highlighted.

While social theorists may have more recently come to cast their critical gaze towards biomedical knowledge, as sociological research into the experience of illness reveals, people who are sick have been doing this for a long time (e.g. Arksey 1994; Garro 1994; Hunt et al. 1989). Within my research, the experiences of women with breast cancer reveal an understanding of the problematics and social constructedness of biomedical knowledge – at least some aspects of biomedical knowledge – even while they simultaneously find comfort, certainty and hope for disease-free lives within biomedicine. One of the places where women articulate this understanding of the social, unstable and politically interested nature of biomedical knowledge is around the issue of breast cancer causation.

Within women's discussions of risk and cause there is a persistent theme that biomedical knowledge about the subject is unstable. This is not surprising if one considers the discourse on breast cancer risk within which women are negotiating their lives with cancer. Debates about the risks posed by high fat diets, alcohol consumption, hormone replacement therapies, birth control pills, environmental carcinogens and many others proliferate. From these discourses one might easily draw the conclusion that *all* knowledge about risks and causes for breast cancer are uncertain and up for debate. Here, a woman describes biomedical knowledge as political, thereby undermining its claim to objectivity and revealing that interests, alliances, and partiality are all part of the construction of biomedical knowledge.

You know, I think that it's a scientific question, but then ultimately it's also a political question ... I think, sort of the path of least resistance is to really focus on the clinical lifestyle factors. What is it about the way that women lead their lives? Do they drink too much ... are they too fat ... do they not exercise enough ... should they be eating less meat? That's ... much more palatable ... It's much easier to say, 'Well you know, alcohol consumption appears to be related to breast cancer and so women really need to think about reducing their alcohol consumption' than saying, 'Gee ... it looks like dioxin may actually be an oestrogenic chemical and may increase the risk of breast cancer.' I mean, we're talking about how we live our lives, our production processes related to everything. And that ... that's politically very contentious.

This particular woman turns the question of why biomedical knowledge is uncertain from a question of what is knowable *scientifically*, to what is knowable *politically*. This questioning of the objectivity of biomedical knowledge is one way that women offer a critique of biomedicine. Another, is the way in which, in the struggle to detect, define and name breast cancer, women's knowledges and biomedical expert knowledges interact and simultaneously produce knowledge. In the following section I draw on the Foucauldian concept of the clinical gaze to explore these ideas.

The Clinical Gaze

In *Birth of a Clinic*, Foucault (1973) argues that disease is socially constructed through the medical gaze. Foucault explores the ways that an historically constituted, rational medical discourse constructs bodies as diseased or not diseased – as pathological or normal. He asserts that medicine constructs disease and illness as phenomena that are located in the body, defined as that which can be reduced, described and articulated through medical discourse. Because the 'truth' of disease is located in the body and the body is defined by medical discourse, it is the sovereign power of the clinical gaze to diagnose, define and control disease. This situation, for Foucault, is historically constructed and socially maintained.

Numerous social theorists have built on Foucault's idea of the social construction of disease through the historically constituted medical gaze. Jackie Orr (1993), for example, offers a critique of Foucauldian theory's tendency to identify disease in its entirety as a biomedical social construction without simultaneously acknowledging other ways that disease may be constructed. She indicates that sociologists must learn from feminists who have suggested 'that while disease may be constituted through the discourse of medicine, it is almost always some "thing" outside its citing by a clinical gaze' (Orr 1993: 452). In acknowledging that disease is also something other than its construction by the clinical gaze, Orr implicates the multiple possibilities for constructing a disease. How one constructs any experience must be understood situationally; for example, an individual experiencing a disease may construct that disease independently of, differently from, or in addition to the construction of the medical gaze. Orr goes on to say of the 'thing' that disease also is outside of its citing by a clinical gaze: 'This "thingness" of disease is not its natural or biological features but its particular relations to the scene in which it materializes as a form, a cultural, economic, symbolic, and gendered scene that includes, but is never restricted to the site of medical practices' (Orr 1993: 452).

The power of the medical gaze to define and articulate breast cancer has consequences for women's own constructions of their embodied illness and the likelihood of that knowledge being taken seriously in the medical encounter. That is, the dominance of the medical gaze as the legitimate producer of knowledges about the body and its diseases means that women's productions of knowledges are often dismissed. It is also true, however, as Orr's assertions reveal, that disease is almost always something outside its citing by the clinical gaze. Breast cancer is experienced and knowledges are constructed about it from multiple sites and draws on multiple sources. As women make sense of their interactions with the medical gaze and simultaneously construct knowledge from other sources, biomedical knowledges are constructed in ways that are both intended and not intended by those doing the constructing. Thus, even in relation to the medical gaze, multiple constructions of knowledge emerge as women negotiate the complex world of biomedicine.

In women's discussions of detection of breast cancer and breast cancer recurrences, there is a tension between the power of the clinical gaze to diagnose and define breast cancer and the simultaneous construction of that knowledge by women through embodied and other knowledge sources. The process that culminates in a breast cancer diagnosis – that is, the process of detection – often begins when a woman senses that something is wrong within her body. This detection is most often based on purely embodied knowledge: the feeling of a small, unusual lump as she is running her hand over her breast in the shower; a sharp pain in her hip as she's walking down the street. Some women find their lumps during a breast self-examination; others find their lumps by accident. This initiation into the process of detection is most often purely embodied and focused on feelings, sensations and knowledges gained through the body. Uncertainty and certainty comingle in women's descriptions of this process. Women often describe an initial 'certainty', but subsequently describe dismissing this certainty or 'putting it out of their head'. Women talk about self-detection in terms of finding 'lumps' not cancer. They do not begin referring to it as their 'cancer' until after a biopsy confers a 'cancer diagnosis'. In this way, embodied knowledge is constructed as uncertain and necessitating 'confirmation' by biomedicine.

Upon detecting cancer at the level of their bodies, women often then turn to their present store of information about breast cancer, whatever that may be. Knowledge may be drawn from experiential resources such as interactions or past experiences with family, friends or other women with breast cancer. For the women who are detecting recurrences this experiential knowledge, of course, includes their own past breast cancer experiences. Women also describe drawing knowledge from information gathered through media or biomedical information gathered from any number of sources.

For example, one woman detected her first recurrence through her embodied experience of a sharp pain in her hip. This then immediately brought to her mind a pamphlet in which she had read about metastatic breast cancer. Upon adding this to her embodied knowledge she was even more convinced that she had a recurrence. In this narrative, the woman captures a way that embodied knowledge is constructed through experiences of pain. This knowledge is then reinforced with biomedical information that she remembered reading in a pamphlet. In the following passage, she illuminates the coexistence of certainty and uncertainty as women derive knowledge of breast cancer detection through embodiment and experience:

> I was walking along one day and I got a pain in my left hip. And I thought, it was an odd thing, but I thought to myself, 'Oh my God, the cancer has come back.' I knew nothing about metastatic breast cancer. I mean nothing. All I had ever read was a little brochure of it given at the time of my diagnosis. And I remember reading in that, it said, 'Unfortunately the prognosis for women with metastatic breast cancer is very poor.' And then it showed a picture of a woman's body and it showed some of the sites where metastases were likely to come and I remember it showed this one thing that's in the hip. And for some reason the minute I felt that pain I said, 'It's come back.' I think I must have been thinking of that picture.

Despite the certainty with which this particular woman describes 'knowing' her cancer had recurred she later goes on to describe dismissing this knowledge by 'putting it out of her mind' until it was legitimated by the 'expert' knowledge of physicians and biotechnology.

Biomedical knowledge is talked about as 'confirming' a woman's embodied knowledge in many of the interviews. Here is how it arose in another story:

> So I found the lump in the summer and it actually was quite large. It felt large. Actually it turned out to be quite large too.

Here, the woman first knows the lump is large according to her body, but it only 'turns out to be large' when she gets it confirmed by biomedicine. She, like the previous woman, highlights the ambiguity associated with knowledge about disease derived from non-biomedical sources. While experientially, embodied and other knowledge sources are meaningful and 'ring true' for women, they also are clearly not a legitimate source of accurate, certain knowledge about the presence of cancer in one's body.

What becomes clear in women's stories is that *how* one knows something places value on *what* it is one can legitimately claim to know. That is, knowing one's cancer through the legitimated, rationalized means prescribed by biomedicine – the clinical and technoscientific gazes of biopsies and mammographies – creates legitimacy for the 'truth' of that knowledge. In contrast, knowing one's cancer through embodiment and experience leads to dismissal of the possibility of certainty about the 'truth' of one's disease.

Within stories of detection and diagnosis women reveal that their knowledge is constructed from multiple sources including the body, biomedical information, 'experts', medical technologies, conversations with other people, and others. As they shift among multiple sources of knowledge women construct different modes of detection as variously certain or uncertain. These constructions of certainty reflect the hierarchical structuring of knowledges and the dominance of that which is associated with science, medicine and technology.

Subjugating Knowledges

A crucial aspect of the multiplicity of knowledges about breast cancer is the unequal distribution of credibility and legitimacy afforded to knowledges derived from different sources. What the women's stories reveal is that certain knowledges are privileged, while others are subjugated in biomedical interactions around breast cancer. Foucault (1980) argues that discourses and texts rationalize and normalize embodied experiences and local situations turning them into a general, standardized knowledge that can be controlled. Thus, knowledge is inextricably linked to power in that the organizations and transmissions of knowledge are ways in which power is exercised. These normalizing discursive processes subjugate certain knowledges and legitimate others. This theory of subjugated knowledge reveals ways in which what comes to be counted as legitimate knowledge in society is replete with power and implicates larger structural forces and social relations in society. It also reveals the corresponding emancipatory potential of knowledge and implicates ideas as sites of resistance and transformation.

Foucault (1980: 81) describes subjugated knowledges as knowledges that are created in conflict or struggle and whose conflict has been erased as these knowledges have been 'buried and disguised in a functionalist coherence or formal systemisation'. Subjugated knowledges include 'a whole set of knowledges that have been disqualified as inadequate to their task or insufficiently elaborated: naïve knowledges, located low down on the hierarchy, beneath the required level of cognition or scientificity' (Foucault, 1980: 82).[2] In the research I conducted, women's knowledges were both implicitly and explicitly dismissed, constructed as naïve and variously subjugated in the hierarchy of knowledges surrounding breast cancer knowledge.

Howard Becker (1967) usefully articulates a 'hierarchy of credibility' in which certain individuals' or groups' claims to knowledge are deemed less credible by virtue of power and position, rather than the content of the knowledge itself. The hierarchy of credibility in knowledges about breast cancer is revealed as women describe which knowledges are 'certain' and which provide 'uncertain' information. In the interviews, the women described seeking mammograms (or other screening technologies in the case of bone metastasis) to confirm what they already sensed in their bodies. Within these narratives, mammography is constructed as a relatively uncertain technology capable of detecting lumps, but not necessarily cancer, while only biopsy provides the certain knowledge of cancer. Certain knowledge, then, is constructed as possible only within a surgical procedure where cancer is actually taken out of the body and tested.

The uncertainty and lack of credibility attributed to experiential knowledge extends not just to women's own embodied experiences, but also to the doctor's. One woman describes this construction well in talking about her doctor's uncertainty that what she was feeling in her breast and what she was seeing on the mammogram was actually cancer:

> She herself didn't think it was anything, but as a smart doctor felt that ultimately one doesn't know what it is until you biopsy it and actually remove it.

In this narrative, the physician was actually feeling the woman's lump with her fingers as well as viewing a representation of the lump on the mammographic film. However, the physician's own embodied knowledge derived through the sensation of her fingers palpating the lump as well as the knowledge she constructed through reading the image on the film were both deemed uncertain. Thus, it is clear that neither women, nor their biomedical practitioners, view all biomedical knowledge equally.

For the women with whom I spoke, only the biopsy is constructed as producing certain knowledge of breast cancer. The biopsy is, itself, not a simple process and some women describe having to have more than one biopsy – a needle aspiration of breast cells and then a surgical removal of breast tissue – before a certain knowledge was achieved. (The processes by which the cells are then analysed and deemed cancerous once they are outside a woman's body is one that women did not address, but which, surely, contains its own processes of negotiations before a breast cancer diagnosis is pronounced.)

In these stories of detection, women's bodies are subjected to technoscientific and biomedical methodologies that attempt to know their bodies and potential disease in a way that many of these women in one way or another 'knew' already through experience. There is a distinct hierarchy of credibility, that is a process from embodied knowledge to mammography to biopsy. While women describe their embodied knowledge as uncertain in many instances, for a significant number it also turned out to be right and so through this first-hand, experientially derived knowledge their cancers were ultimately detected. In a sense a demystification of dominant ways of knowing occurs. This demystification is reinforced in stories that women told about detection failures and breast cancer that was inadvertently detected. Here, embodied knowledge turned out to be more reliable for many women who subsequently describe experiences of technological and biomedical failures.

All the women I interviewed had stories to tell about uncertain biomedical knowledge in relationship to detection. In this way, detection turned out to be a significant site in which biomedical constructions of breast cancer were disrupted. Women related tales of biomedical and technoscientific mistakes and near-misses. These tales included detection that occurred inadvertently while other procedures were taking place upon a woman's body, either related or not, and tumours that were perpetually undetectable through the means of biomedicine.

A compelling aspect of these stories is that failures and mistakes were often only counteracted by women's assertions of their embodied knowledges. For example, one woman told the following story:

> I had a palpable mass, at least palpable for me for the last two years. And they could not detect anything on mammography. And so this year I scheduled an appointment with my gynaecologist early and ... I should preface all of this with the fact that I have bilateral implants. And ... my gynaecologist felt that it was an edge of the implant that I was palpating. And this year I said, there is definitely something ... I could feel where it started, but not where it ended and had my mammograms early this year and again they reassured me that everything was fine and that they were the same as last year. And I insisted that it was not fine and I went to speak to the radiologist which ended up being a bit of a confrontation. He tried to reassure me that everything was OK. My mammograms were clear and ... I insisted that he palpate this area and I was not comfortable in leaving and waiting for another year. Finally in this struggle, they agreed to do some spot magnifications basically to relieve my anxiety. And he came back shortly and said on the magnification there was a spiculated mass that looked malignant, certainly should be investigated. It took me a bit of time to get a surgeon and he put the mammogram over the light and said, 'You know there's better than a 90 per cent chance that this is malignant. But, it looks like a small tumour, And so, after my biopsy he did find out that it was a ductal invasive.

In this story, the woman's intimate experience of her own body is actively dismissed as a reliable source of knowledge. It is only after her struggle with the radiologist that her embodied knowledge is taken into account. Ultimately, as in most detection trajectories, certain knowledge of her cancer was only arrived at through the biopsy. Her story provides a powerful critique of the technologies, biomedical practitioners and procedures that, despite their uncertainties, are placed above individual experiences in the hierarchy of credible knowledges about breast cancer.

Several of the women's experiences address biomedical uncertainty in that their cancer was coincidentally detected while they were undergoing another procedure. Within these stories, there is the clear implication that the detection occurred by 'accident' and that the cancer could have just as easily *not* been detected. For example, in the following narrative, a woman describes the detection of her breast cancer occurring inadvertently when her surgeon was performing a biopsy on something else that turned out not to be cancer.

> So, in March of '94 I had my first biopsy. And when they went in ... what they took out showed the calcification was nothing ... But in the tissue near the calcification they found a cluster ... of cancer.

In this story, the original calcification was detected through a mammogram. Here, biomedical knowledge is constructed as uncertain because of its failure to detect that which was indeed cancerous, as well as its mistaken detection of something that was not. To have both those mistakes within the same procedure creates a sense of randomness about whether cancer is or is not detected by biomedical technologies like mammography.

Another woman also describes an experience with biomedicine in which her cancer was inadvertently detected. In her case, a second primary tumour was found in her breast, which had previously been thought to be non-cancerous when she had it removed prophylactically. She had already had mammograms on both breasts in response to the lump she had felt in the breast; both a mammogram and biopsy subsequently detected and confirmed this to be cancerous. This second tumour did not show up on any of the tests she had had up to that point:

> I decided to have the other breast removed prophylactically and also for cosmetic reasons and when they did that they found a second primary in the second breast that didn't show up on any test, mammogram, anything.

Similar to the previous story, this narrative highlights the seeming randomness that some cancers can be detected through mammograms, self-examinations and other tests, while others cannot. The relief at having detected the second breast cancer is tempered by the awareness that biomedical detection technologies are not the certain, unproblematic methods that they are often touted to be.

Finally, one woman describes the unintentional detection of her recurrence in this excerpt:

> I have a herniated disc and it was giving me a lot of problems and I went to an orthopaedic surgeon who did X-rays and MRIs and when I went back to see him he said ... 'There is this spot on your pelvis and, you know I don't think we can go ahead with any treatment for your back until we find out what it is.' I had a bone biopsy and it turned out to be an oestrogen-receptive breast cancer.

The randomness of this detection left this woman with a sense of the unknowability of cancer, its hidden presence in the body and a sense that detection was a fortunate mistake, a mistake that could have easily not occurred:

> I don't have any pain ... I would never have known at this point that I had this tumour if I hadn't had the MRI and X-rays for the back pain. You know, it's just a hidden thing that ... that's there and who knows.

In this excerpt, the woman eloquently captures the fundamental uncertainty of cancer. She highlights the absence of pain or other embodied markers and thus the seeming hiddenness of cancer within the body. It is precisely this hiddenness that technoscientific imaging devices such as mammography and MRI are supposed to transcend. However, as these women's stories reveal, that transcendence cannot be relied on, as the images that are captured do not necessarily reveal the presence or absence of cancer in the body.

Again, women's accounts reveal a demystification of dominant ways of knowing as they assert fundamental uncertainties and potential failings pertaining to these ways of knowing that in dominant discourse are seen as better and most reliable. By starting with women's experience and taking seriously women's knowledge these hierarchies are problematized and critiqued.

Bifurcated Consciousness

Women's knowledges of breast cancer, grounded as they are in lived experience, provide a critique of discursive and textually mediated expert biomedical knowledge. This critique emerges at the rupture that often exists between that which is known through lived experience and that which is disseminated as breast cancer knowledge by experts, and illustrates Dorothy Smith's theories of a feminist sociology of knowledge (Smith 1990). For Smith, knowledge is intimately linked with the 'practices of power' because it is through knowledge that the relations of ruling dominate, and also through knowledge that critique and resistance to domination emerge. She also describes how power is affirmed when knowledge is disseminated vis-à-vis texts – a process we can see at work in relation to women's constructions of knowledge of breast cancer, where the dominant, biomedical knowledge disseminated about breast cancer is often accomplished through texts. This is one of the reasons why conceptualizing the interactions between women and biomedical knowledges as occurring 'inside' or 'outside' biomedicine is problematic. Instead, the proliferation of biomedical expert knowledge mediated through texts means that the spaces in which women negotiate biomedical knowledge and construct their own biomedical knowledge occur neither within nor without biomedicine. The consequences of textually mediated knowledges described by Smith, and which reveal the connections between power and knowledge, provide a useful analytical framework for understanding the processes at work in this particular situation.

In contemporary society, according to Smith (1990), our knowledge is increasingly mediated by texts. There is a way of knowing that is grounded in our everyday experience and, simultaneously, a way of knowing that we come to through texts. Those with power in society construct and transmit certain knowledges that legitimate and accomplish their positions of power. These knowledges come to be the dominant and taken-for-granted knowledges about what is 'true' and 'real' in society. At the same time, knowledge emerges through embodied experiences. The relations of ruling transform these embodied 'everyday and everynight' experiences, and the knowledges that emerge from them, into abstract, textual knowledge as a means of control. Experience thus normalized and rationalized is drawn into a controllable realm wherein the relations of ruling can most efficiently rule. The usefulness of abstract, textual knowledges to the relations of ruling means that they end up being the most validated and legitimized knowledge. Within this scheme, personal experience is discarded as a reliable source of information. 'Issues are formulated because they are administratively relevant, not because they are significant first in the experience of those who live them' (Smith 1990: 15).

According to Smith, this way of conceptualizing knowledge for the purposes of ruling 'establishes two modes of knowing and experiencing and doing, one located in the body and in the space it occupies and moves in, the other ... passing beyond the local into the conceptual order' (Smith, 1990: 17). For those who maintain an active consciousness in both modes of knowing, a bifurcation of consciousness exists. From this bifurcation a critical standpoint emerges. On the one hand, women receive knowledge that reflects the experiences of those in power. Yet, on the other hand, this knowledge is often contrary to the knowledges emerging out of their own experiences and interactions in their everyday worlds. Women are thus in a unique position to critique the dominant system as they maintain an awareness of the disjuncture between the knowledges produced by those who rule and the everyday knowledges produced in material existence. In my project, women can be seen as occupying this critical position of bifurcation and constructing knowledges that reveal the spaces that exist between that which biomedicine disseminates as knowledge about breast cancer and those knowledges that are meaningful to the lives of women living with the disease.

Women's knowledges and experiences emerge as a critique of discursive and textually mediated expert knowledges about breast cancer most clearly in their critiques of discourses of early detection. The demystification of dominant ways of knowing that women accomplish through their detection narratives is seen explicitly in their direct critiques of biomedical knowledges of early detection and the dissemination of biomedical discourses of early detection. Both breast self-examination and mammography are problematized as well as the larger discourse that early detection is prevention.

While most of the women I talked to discovered their own lumps, this embodied knowledge was seldom derived from the biomedically approved method of breast self-examination. A couple of the women talked about doing breast self-examination before their diagnosis, but this process is described as problematic and imbued with uncertainties. For example, one woman relates:

> I knew about breast self-exam and mammograms and that those
> were good things to do. But, you know, you really don't realize the

implications of what it means when you get bombarded constantly about the *need* to do breast self-exams and the *need* to do mammograms ... I never gave any thought to the implications of that. One of which is it gives a false impression that breast self-exam is like a preventative measure, which it isn't. It's not. It's not preventative. It doesn't prevent you from getting breast cancer.

In this narrative, biomedical knowledge about what constitutes appropriate health strategies is not seen as neutral and unproblematically beneficial. Rather, this woman reveals the implications of this knowledge, of its dominance and proliferation. She describes the way in which it conflates what is a detection practice with actual prevention. In another excerpt, she draws attention to a further implication of the biomedical knowledge about early detection and breast self-exam as shifting the responsibility for detection away from biomedicine and on to women themselves – a process that leads to blaming women for their own disease. She says:

[It's] a very controversial issue too to trash breast self-exam 'cause it is one of the few things women have. And I would never trash it. But ... it basically puts the onus on women to detect their cancer. And it basically implies if you haven't been ... doing the search and destroy mission on your boob every month and you have breast cancer and it's advanced then it's basically your fault ... It takes sort of the onus away from the medical community.

Another woman makes similar critiques about the conflation of early detection and prevention but here in relation to mammography. She says:

... the news guy writes this op. ed. piece ... his second wife died of breast cancer. And ... he's talking about mammography as prevention. And ... he talks about this woman who heard his public service announcement about breast cancer. This woman heard it – she'd been putting off having her mammogram – she goes and has it and she found out that she has breast cancer. [reading from article] 'It turns out that early detection saved her life.' *Baloney!!* [laughing] I'm going to write to the [paper]. The myth that mammography somehow equals prevention is out there.

Here, the source of knowledge that she specifically points to is popular media and its coverage of biomedical discourses.

Women's critiques of mammograms as an unproblematic detection behaviour extend to include consideration of the risk that one undergoes by irradiating their breasts once a year. One woman captures this well:

> Mammograms [are] touted as this incredibly wonderful thing . . . you know, and women should always get their mammograms and then there was a debate whether or not it was after forty after fifty blah blah blah blah. But, basically, if you got your mammograms you were safe. And . . . no discussion about the trade-off of irradiating your breast every year for instance. Or in my case . . . obviously . . . I'm gonna get one every year now but, you know, I do think about it. It's like, OK, well I'm gonna irradiate my breast every year since the age 28. I mean, you know, that's probably going to ultimately be a problem. Of course, I would not not do it. But, you know, it's like you don't really . . . I didn't have as acute awareness of how problematic these things are until I actually had to go through it myself and gave it some thought.

Radiation is the only currently known cause of breast cancer and this narrative highlights the problematic irony that the best screening technology for the detection of breast cancer relies on the carcinogenic properties of radiation.

This woman also reveals a fundamental issue for many women as they negotiate biomedical constructions of breast cancer, and why beginning with their lived experiences provides such valuable critique and insight: that one does not have an awareness of how problematic biomedical constructions of knowledge are until one is actually experiencing breast cancer. Because these women are most aware of the ways that dominant biomedical discourse does and does not reflect the actualities of the experience of breast cancer, it is by highlighting their constructions of knowledge that a particularly useful critique can emerge. The critique of dominant biomedical discourses also emerged in the bifurcation between women's experiences of 'cure' and dominant discourses about 'cure'.

'Cure' is part of the discourse that is transmitted to women about the disease of breast cancer. It is talked about by biomedical experts as a possibility for women whose breast cancer is detected early enough and treated properly. The problematics of this discourse are clear to the women with whom I spoke. One woman relates a story that encapsulates the biomedical discourse of cure as framed by an 'expert':

> It's interesting I'm working on this film …[and] I had the *distinct pleasure* of interviewing NIH scientists …and … I asked [one of the scientists] if … breast cancer had touched her in any personal way and she said, 'Yes I'm a survivor and I've been out for five years and breast cancer's a curable disease.' Which I thought was unbelievable coming from a scientist telling me that. And [she also said], that 'I eat well and work out and don't eat meat anymore and I've changed my lifestyle and for that reason I'm not going to get it anymore.' And so the message is that women have control over this.

In this discourse, not only is breast cancer constructed as curable but also as the personal responsibility of women with the disease to make sure they are cured. Another woman also describes being told that breast cancer is curable, this time in relation to her own disease:

> So I was given an *excellent* prognosis. Really, they had every expectation that the mastectomy had cured me of cancer.

For this woman, this prognosis of 'cure' was disrupted six months after it was conferred when she had her first recurrence and has continued to be disrupted as she is now dying of the breast cancer which was supposedly 'cured' seven years ago. Other women, too, describe coming to realize through their own experience and the experiences of those around them that 'breast cancer is not a curable disease'. From these experiences, women construct breast cancer as something that one never is cured from. One woman relates:

> And the hardest part about having the recurrence is that I used to say, 'I *had* cancer.' And I've learned now that you can *never* say, 'I had cancer.'

This woman had a recurrence 15 years after her original diagnosis and thus, she took great issue with the dominant construction of five-year, disease-free survival rates equalling cure.

Another woman's construction of 'cure' was disrupted by watching those around her die of breast cancer. Her narrative highlights the extreme uncertainty of breast cancer: you only know 'that you're not going to die of breast cancer' when 'you're dying of something else':

I guess I always had before viewed breast cancer as something that you could definitely recover from. And if you discover it early you'll get better which is sometimes the case, but sometimes it's not. And you really realize that sometimes it's not when you're the one who gets it. You know when you start going to breast cancer groups and women around you start getting recurrences and it's like a real eye-opener ... That some people don't get better and they die. And they die a slow and very painful death and that's very scary especially when you're twenty-eight years old and you figure you have a long time before you become an old lady. And you have a long time before you discover that ... you know, you really don't know that you're not going to die of breast cancer until you're dying of something else.

What this quote so eloquently reveals is the way that lived experience as a source of knowledge disrupts and problematizes dominant, biomedical knowledge constructions about breast cancer in extremely important ways. There is an interaction between dominant discourses about breast cancer and personal experience that can reveal both the nuances of the experiences of breast cancer as well as its position within larger social structural relations in society. In this way, women's voices and experiences provide a powerful critique and tool for social change.

Conclusion

In conclusion, this chapter captures some of the complex interactions and knowledge constructions that take place as women negotiate the biomedical world of breast cancer. These biomedically defined aspects of women's experiences of breast cancer are a few of the multiple arenas in which breast cancer is lived and knowledge of breast cancer is constructed. I have focused on them as important sites to explore the convergence of lived experience, biomedical discourse and the resulting construction of biomedicine as contestable and problematic. I have explored the way that biomedicine and the technoscientific gaze confer legitimacy and construct legitimate knowledges. Such an interrogation reveals *how* what is known shapes the values placed on *what* is known. At the same time, experientially, women describe how biomedicine and its technologies can and do fail, and thus the knowledge they produce becomes uncertain and problematic. Women experiencing breast cancer are in a uniquely privileged position to construct a critique of biomedicine that illuminates the disruption between discourse and experience. From this critique, we should learn strategies for producing knowledges that can better heal the many wounds inflicted by breast cancer by drawing on lived, embodied experiences, emotions, and other previously dismissed and suppressed sources of knowledge.

Notes

1 For example, emotional experience is one source that women described drawing on to construct knowledge about their disease. Despite the representation of emotion as a thoroughly delegitimate, irrational (and thus the opposite of objective truth) source of knowledge, it never the less is described by women as a source for constructing knowledge about breast cancer.
2 Patricia Hill Collins (1991) takes issue with Foucault's description of subjugated knowledges as naïve. In my mind, subjugated knowledges are constructed as naïve by virtue of their position as subjugated. The process of suppressing certain knowledges involves constructing them in opposition to whatever counts as legitimate knowledge.

References

Arksey, H. 'Expert and Lay Participation in the Construction of Medical Knowledge'. *Sociology of Health and Illness* 16 (1994) pp. 448–68.
Becker, H. 'Whose Side Are We On?' *Social Problems* 14 (1967) pp. 239–47.
Estes, C. and Binney, E. 'The Biomedicalization of Aging: Dangers and Dilemmas'. *The Gerontologist* 29 (1989) pp. 587–96.
Foucault, M. *Power/Knowledge: Selected Interviews and Other Writings* (New York: Pantheon Books 1980).
Foucault, M. *Birth of a Clinic* (New York: Tavistock Publications 1973).
Garro, L. 'Narrative Representations of Chronic Illness Experience: Cultural Models of Illness, Mind and Body in Stories Concerning the Temporomandibular Joint (TMJ)'. *Social Science and Medicine* 38 (1994) pp. 775–88.
Hunt, L., B. Jordon and S. Irwin. 'Views of What's Wrong: Diagnosis and Patients' Concepts of Illness'. *Social Science and Medicine* 28 (1989) pp.945–56.
Lock, M. and P. Kaufert, eds. *Pragmatic Women and Body Politics* (Cambridge: Cambridge University Press 1988).
Lock, M. and D. Gordon, eds. *Biomedicine Examined* (Boston: Kluwer Academic Publishers 1988).
Mannheim, K. *Essays on the Sociology of Knowledge*, ed. Paul Kecskemeti. (London: Routledge, 1952).
Orr, J. 'Panic Diaries: (Re)Constructing a Partial Politics and Poetics of Disease'. In Holstein, J. and G. Miller, eds. *Reconsidering Social Constructionism: Debates in Social Problems Theory* (New York: Aldine DeGruyter 1993).
Smith, D. *The Conceptual Practices of Power: A Feminist Sociology of Knowledge.* (Boston: Northeastern University Press 1990).

Strauss, A. and J. Corbin. *Basics of Qualitative Research: Grounded Theory Procedures and Techniques* (London: Sage Publications 1990).

Ward, S. *Reconfiguring Truth, Postmodernism, Science Studies, and the Search for a New Model of Knowledge* (Lanham: Rowman & Littlefield Publishers 1996).

Wright, P. and A. Treacher. *The Problem of Medical Knowledge* (Edinburgh: Edinburgh University Press 1982).

2
Sexualized Illness: the Newsworthy Body in Media Representations of Breast Cancer

Cherise Saywell, with Lisa Beattie and Lesley Henderson

Breast cancer is unusual among illnesses, especially among other cancers, because of the specific ways that its bodily site – the female breast – is sexualized in popular representations. Illness, particularly cancer, has historically been shrouded in suspicion and fear, expressed through taboos and via euphemisms. Femininity, in its maternal and sexual manifestations, is frequently situated as passive and body-centred in dominant discourses. Cultural anxieties about breast cancer are determined by the intersection of popular discourses of femininity and illness at the icon of the breast, and complicated by its status as diseased. Taboos of illness and cancer are veiled by the erotic potential of the fetishized breast, and subjects are referenced according to gendered discourses which situate them according to discourses of sexual and maternal femininity.

This chapter demonstrates this in an analysis of press coverage of breast cancer in the UK. It draws on a study into the production, reception and content of media representations of breast cancer and focuses on how the British news media depict women with breast cancer.[1] The media are a rich site for exploring representations of breast cancer. Health issues – historically the province of the private realm and traditionally a 'women's issue' – have become increasingly visible as news in recent years. Health issues have migrated from women's magazines to the more public domain of daily newspapers, as part of 'health pages', news pages, and even featured on the front page. Breast cancer in particular has received steadily increasing coverage in recent years[2] and it is currently the most visible cancer in press coverage of health. Its media profile is higher than that of all other common cancers.[3] For example, breast cancer was headlined seven times more frequently than lung cancer between 1995 and 1997, despite recent evidence which shows lung cancer kills almost as many women. Indeed, in Scotland lung cancer has a higher mortality rate than breast cancer (Cancer Research Campaign 1996). The following analysis is based on a study of three years' press coverage comprising three daily broadsheets (*The Guardian, The Independent* and *The Times*), two daily tabloids (*The Sun* and *The Mirror*) and three broadsheet Sunday newspapers (*The Observer, The Independent* and *The Sunday Times*), all of which are UK national newspapers.

Women's bodies, especially young women's bodies, make breast cancer newsworthy. This can be seen in both the imagery and narratives which construct media representations of breast cancer. First, the iconography of breast cancer is structured by images of the fetishized and idealized youthful breast. The 'sexiness' of breasts is used to 'sell' breast cancer. Correspondingly, mastectomies are constructed as, above all, a violation of femininity. This preoccupation is ascribed through media focus on youthful sufferers of breast cancer. Thus while the illness is experienced primarily by menopausal women, its representatives in the press are comparatively younger. Their narratives are centred on myths of tragic motherhood and triumphant sacrifice, and their losses are situated in terms of mutilated femininity. The final section of this chapter explores how breast cancer might be represented in different ways by exploring some accounts which diverge from these norms.

Whose Breast? Situating the Breast in Breast Cancer

Breast cancer is framed by cultural understandings and conceptions of illness, traditionally marked by anxiety and encased in metaphor. Cancer is viewed with particular horror in Western cultures (Sontag 1978; Stacey 1997). While other illnesses are deadly, humiliating and/or painful, few carry the connotations or particular dread that cancer does (Stacey, 1997: 73). Jackie Stacey argues that this is partly because cancer challenges our understanding of the body in terms of its vulnerability, its integrity and its potential for violation. She says that 'the body has been understood to be constituted within and through a system of boundaries, which are integral to wider beliefs about defilement and purification' (Stacey 1997: 75). Cancer violates these boundaries, generating anxieties about the certainty of boundaries between subject and object, normal and abnormal, inside and outside, and between life and death (Stacey 1997: 77). For example, while cells are life-giving, and cell division marks the very beginning of life, cancer is caused by this process accelerating out of control. It is a disease of uncontrolled life whereby the boundaries between life and death are unrecognizable. The malignant cell originates within, and is produced by, the body. It is often conceptualized and even personified as deceptive, because the cancer hides inside, protects itself: 'it impersonates the subject long enough to establish the power of its real difference, often until it can overpower its host body' (Stacey 1997: 78). Diagnosis usually occurs well after the cancer has taken hold of the body.

Cancer is, additionally, described as a grotesque disease because of its potential for mutilation and violation, and its ability to permeate bodily boundaries. For example, tumours are formed from bodily matter and are part of the organs they originate from. However, they can enlarge these organs and transgress boundaries separating inside from outside by protruding from the body and even breaking through the skin. Treatment for cancer kills healthy cells in order to destroy the cancerous ones, and chemotherapy, while suppressing the illness, causes nausea and vomiting, hair loss and infertility.

Cancer historically has been surrounded by strenuous conventions of concealment. This is motivated by a public sense of horror at cancer which is embedded in metaphors, innuendo and euphemism through which it is conceptualized and spoken; for example, in the UK, a well-known euphemism for cancer is 'The Big C'. Its language is constructed by the cultural anxiety which surrounds it, and sanitized by the silences which cushion its particular horror. Like other illnesses, breast cancer is constructed through the disavowals, absences and denials of meaning which surround sickness in general and cancer in particular. However, breast cancer is especially culturally laden because of the problematic ways in which femininity is located in and value attributed to the female body. Western cultures idealize femininity as passive and bodily centred. Women are attributed value via bodies which are sexualized and commodified for the male gaze and masculine consumption; or through bodies which are conceptualized in terms of reproductive potential.

Breasts are iconic both of female sexuality and maternity, and as such, are often the currency through which feminine value is attributed. This is particularly visible and visual, in the representation of the erotic breast. Taboos on exposure add layers of sexual connotation to the breast. Breasts function as women's 'sexual ornaments – the crown jewels of femininity' (Yalom, 1997: 3). However in their sexual function, they are concealed, revealed, adorned and exhibited primarily for and from a male point of view. This is evident from Renaissance art, which first sexualized and eroticized this aspect of female anatomy in the West, to page 3 pin ups.

The maternal breast is no less idealized, but is marked by its distance from its eroticized counterpart. While both represent an idealized version of femininity, they are wholly separate manifestations. Breasts in their maternal function made the news (in an article titled in rather unsubtle fashion, 'Knockers Slate New Breast Ads', *The Sun*, 27 December 1997, p. 38), in response to promotional images of breast feeding, which were perceived to be too sexy. The advertisement was slated for too closely merging the sexual and maternal functions of the breast. The breast photographed was criticized for being too pert and the soft-focused image too sexy for a maternal representation. The write-up in *The Sun* evidences the conventional separation of maternal and sexual breasts through use of desexualizing terminology. The lactating breast is described using terms like 'mammaries', 'udder' 'milking machine' and 'milk production'.

In relation to breast cancer, Alisa Solomon states that 'because it occurs in that iconic lump of flesh – both erotic and maternal – [breast cancer] brings the sexism in women's health issues to the surface' (1995: 158). The 'cancerous' breast can be neither erotic nor maternal, but is constantly situated in relation to either or both of these dominant discourses of femininity. This is especially evident in the media preoccupation with breast cancer. While breast cancer coverage is influenced by the organization of news sources and feminist and women's interest agendas, it is also structured by the public fascination which breast cancer holds. Luisa Dillner, medical columnist for *The Guardian*, encapsulates this, describing breast cancer as 'in news terms' a 'sexy disease' (14 January 1997). In media representations of breast cancer, the breast is framed in terms of its sexual potential. This is exemplified in the disproportionate representation of young women in media coverage: breast cancer reporting is heavily preoccupied with youthful breasts, only occasionally focusing on the menopausal breasts most frequently affected.

In many ways, the menopausal breast is already situated outside the sexual/maternal dichotomy discussed above. Menopause, marking the end of menstruation, is medicalized and pathologized in Western cultures. Women are rarely constructed as normative sexual beings during or after menopause. It is often situated as a 'life of living decay' (Voda 1993: 448) and largely described in terms of loss: 'loss of reproductive ability of hormones, of youth, of bones, of sexuality' (Voda

1993: 451). The cessation of reproductive potential parallels the view of menopause as the twilight of women's sexual lives (in fact, the end of menstruation might represent a kind of sexual freedom for some women, in that sex might be indulged in without the threat of unwanted pregnancy), while the breast, perhaps the most visible symbol of sexual appeal and maternal potential, is culturally devalued after menopause.

Breast cancer reporting reflects this in its focus on young women's bodies. Examination of newspaper reporting on breast cancer reveals a marked gap between the demographic/epidemiological reality of breast cancer and the cancer victims/survivors represented in media accounts. In reality most women who get breast cancer are past their menopause: of the 34,000 diagnoses in the UK each year, only 7,000 are pre-menopausal (CRC Institute for Cancer Studies 1997). However, most 'ordinary' women with breast cancer represented in the above press sample were young women. Where age was indicated 85 per cent were under 50, and of these 38 per cent were 35 or under. (In 20 per cent of cases, no age was mentioned.)[4] In addition, almost half the articles featuring an ordinary breast cancer survivor/victim referenced the sexuality or attractiveness of the subject (most frequently in the case of younger survivors).

This is also reflected in the kinds of images which accompany breast cancer reporting and consistently present readers with images of young and healthy breasts – either full and voluptuous, or young and pert. Images of self-examination exemplify this, showing young women, whether photographed or drawn. Eyes closed, arm raised, hand on breast – these images allude to eroticized, as well as medicalized, discourses. Similarly, newspaper images of mammography screening typically employ young women's bodies even though breast screening is most pertinent as an issue for women in the post-menopausal age bracket (50–65).[5] That said, images of mammography screening are far more likely to employ older women as visual subjects than are depictions of self-examination. This is especially the case in television news coverage where subjects filmed are often older women. However, this tendency could be read as culturally 'safe' within the erotic/maternal framework. Medical imaging does not harbour any of the erotic potential that self-examination might; thus a post-menopausal body can readily be medicalised and 'de-sexualised'.

This overt sexualizing of illness sites separates breast cancer from other cancers, such as bowel cancer. One press officer interviewed as part of the above project stated this outright:

Breasts have a social significance, sexual significance as well. It's not going to make the best magazine with pictures of bowels ... and colostomies are hardly the sort of stuff catwalk models are going to get involved in whereas breast cancer is in the media sense and in a social sense a much more sexy subject. (Henderson 1997)

Lisa Cartwright writes of a conjunction between fashion and breast cancer in the US (1998: 122). The same could be said of the marketing of breast cancer in the UK, which is similarly built up around breasts which are imaged as icon and fetish object, and is correspondingly reliant on images of youthful femininity for this. Breast cancer campaigns attract the support of young, attractive, celebrity patrons who lend their names and bodies (and their healthy breasts) to it as a cause. Supermodel Claudia Schiffer, celebrity model Sophie Dahl and Wonderbra girl Eva Herzigova feature in reports about breast cancer with headlines like 'Girls Go to War' (*Scottish Mirror*, 24 April 1996), 'It's a bra-illiant idea' (*Scottish Mirror*, 11 June 1997) and 'Hello Girls' (*Scottish Mirror*, 9 October 1996). The latter headline is a play on Herzigova's well-known Wonderbra campaign caption, 'Hello Boys'.

The exploitation of the media's attraction to the (healthy) breast is encouraged by some fund-raising activities. Breast cancer made the front page of *The Sun* following the London Marathon (27 April 1998), when the race was run by women wearing Wonderbras to raise money for research. Television celebrity Julia Carling was pictured wearing a customized Wonderbra, and described as preparing to 'breast the tape' following the race. The 'body pun' which accompanied the Julia Carling image is typical of a lot of breast cancer reporting, illustrating a cultural preoccupation with the bodily site of the illness. Headlines are replete with such innuendo, evidencing the very particular threat of breast surgery. Body 'puns' play on what is at stake in an unsubtle way, as in the following headlines:

'The Unbearable Naked Truth' (*The Guardian*, 16 April 1996)

'Keeping Abreast of Breast Cancer' (*The Guardian*, 9 September 1995)

'Beast in the Breast' (*The Guardian*, 29 October 1996)

'The Breast Option' (*The Sun*, 10 January 1996)

'Beauty and the Breast' (*The Guardian*, 3 October 1995)

The Absent Breast – Mastectomies in the Media

Contrasting with the plentiful breast images accompanying breast cancer stories, images of mastectomy are rare. In the three-year newspaper sample underlying this study, involving nearly 800 items, there were only two pictures of mastectomized breasts.[6] One image was from a Vegetarian Society advertisement and pictured three scars, one of which represents a mastectomy scar. The advertisement was the second most complained about that year (An Ad Too Far From the Tofu & Muesli Merchants, 19 October 1997). The only other image of a mastectomized chest was a photograph of a mastectomy scar on a man who had had breast cancer (*Daily Mirror,* 20 March 1995).

This absence speaks loudly about meanings surrounding mastectomy. Like other forms of amputation, perceptions of mastectomy and lumpectomy are governed by ideas about disfigurement, damage and mutilation. Its associations are with disease and not recovery. Broadly, the absent breast is a signifier of those cultural taboos discussed earlier, which surround cancer. Amputation is primarily associated with cancer in the popular consciousness because treatment often involves partial or entire removal of organs affected. Not many other modern illnesses are so consistently linked to ideas about mutilation.

However, because the breast iconicizes images of idealized femininity, the asymmetry of mastectomy and lumpectomy represents an assault on beauty and perceptions of normality. The missing or mutilated breast is referenced according to its distance from what has been called 'the Official Breast' – pert, firm and high, it is a reassuring guarantee of extreme youth (Naomi Wolf, cited in Brooks 1998: 32). Dimpling, puckering or missing breast tissue, like those signifiers of age – sagging, weight gain, etc. – represent aspects of female bodily transformation that are held in general public contempt (Cartwright 1998: 133). Mastectomy is perceived to be a violation of femininity within this paradigm, and is generally hidden and treated as a source of shame.

Thus, as Jackie Stacey emphasizes, the processes surrounding mastectomy and post-operative recovery are designed to reaffirm and reproduce sexual and gender identities. 'To keep one's femininity intact requires elaborate efforts on the part of the woman with cancer: above all, energy should be directed into covering up the signs of this stigmatised disease and the effects of its treatments' (Stacey 1997: 71). She cites Eve Kozofsky Sedgewick, an academic, who speaks from her experience of breast cancer, drawing attention to the rituals surrounding recovery: 'with the proper toning exercise, make-up, wigs and a well-fitting prosthesis, we could feel just as feminine as we ever had and no one (ie. no man) need ever know that anything had happened' (*ibid.* 71). This is affirmed in the kinds of representations of post-mastectomy subjects in the above media sample. Both tabloid and broadsheet newspapers tend to focus disproportionately on the impact of the loss of a breast on femininity and body image. Recovery is signified by a 'recovered' feminine form, and where this is not the case, evidence of loss is concealed.

The media accounts discussed above reproduce these ideas, especially visually. The kinds of post-operative images of women which feature in personal accounts emphasize this recovery of norms of femininity. Most women pictured are symmetrically reconstructed, or conceal the evidence of illness. For example, in '17 in My Family Have Died from Breast Cancer', subject Jayne is pictured post-(prophylactic) mastectomy, full breasted, with just a hint of her bra showing through her blouse (*Scottish Mirror* 9 October 1996). In 'I Partied My Way through Chemo' (*The Sun,* 8 October 1997) Maria is pictured celebrating the end of her treatment wearing a bikini on a beach, and sitting bra-less in a summer dress, visually unscathed by surgery. Where visual references to mastectomy occur, they are commonly depersonalized and/or medicalized with subjects being photographed below the neck, or with their faces blanked out (Cartwright 1998: 133). Images might be framed more overtly by assumptions of body horror, playing directly on cultural fear of the grotesque body described earlier.

This was the case in one image located outside the three-year sample underlying this study. The comparative rarity of images of mastectomies prompted a search outside the original study remit, and yielded a Scottish press front-page feature called 'Breast Op Doc Made Me a Freak' (*Daily Record,* 10 April 1997). The article recounts an extreme story about reconstructive surgery, situating the procedure firmly within discourses of body horror. The piece is accompanied by a sub-heading 'The shocking picture Josephine Day wanted the world to see'. The emphasis on Josephine's desire for the world to see the image reinforces perceptions that it is not a 'tasteful' subject matter (even for a tabloid). She is pictured, naked to the waist, looking docilely at the camera. The story is littered with Frankensteinian metaphors which play on the violation of femininity. The misshapenness of the breasts is explicitly described. This plays on cultural fears about violated bodies as 'leaky vessels' (where fluids break bodily boundaries – commonly associated with the anti-ideal of the feminine body) and about malformation, where body parts are not where they should be – a sense of horror is accentuated in the case of sexual organs:

> Every morning and evening, Josephine Day looks in horror at her once-attractive body. Like something out of a horror film, the nipple of her left breast sits near the centre of her chest ... Her other breast has collapsed completely – its contents oozed out from under her arm after the operation ... 'My poor family were totally traumatised when they saw my leaking wounds and the livid purple scarring from hip to hip ... There was a smell coming from my wounds – like rotten meat. Nothing I did could get rid of it.'

None of the above constitutes an argument against the fact that mastectomy and surgical reconstruction are traumatic experiences. Nor does it deny Josephine's anger. However, accounts like this, because of the way in which they are featured, and because they are rare, reinforce the particular horror of mastectomy. In this framework, there is no positive angle from which women can begin to perceive themselves as whole, as recovering or surviving. Mastectomy can only be understood as mutilatory, and mutilatory in a profound and special sense that must be hidden from the world.

Cancer Narratives

Narratives about breast cancer function similarly, situating the illness within trajectories of life-events whereby feminine worth is determined in sexual and maternal terms and threatened by the diseased breast. This can be seen in an examination of two major sub-genres of breast cancer reporting which focus on prophylactic mastectomies and mothers with breast cancer.

Stories about prophylactic mastectomy – breast removal to reduce the likelihood of development of cancer – formed a substantial sub-genre within breast cancer reporting. These stories explored women's experiences of seeking mastectomies in the face of a high inherited risk and fears of having 'the breast cancer gene'. Women who develop breast cancer as a result of having the breast cancer gene (BRCA1 or BRCA2) form a small minority of breast cancer sufferers. Between 5 and 10 per cent of women with breast cancer have a genetic mutation (Yalom 1997: 233). Most subjects reported within this sub-genre of breast cancer coverage had not developed breast cancer but were part of 'cancer-dense' families where many female relatives had had cancer.

The following headlines, among others, focused on women in 'cancer-dense' families undergoing prophylactic mastectomy:

'17 in My Family Have Died from Breast Cancer' (*Scottish Mirror*, 9 October 1996)

'The Breast Cancer Family' (*The Observer*, 30 June 1996)

'9 of My Family Got Cancer so I Had My Breasts Removed in Case I Was the Next' (*Scottish Mirror*, 14 February 1996)

'Cutting Deadly Odds' (*Scottish Mirror*, 29 May 1996)

These stories play on the cultural horror of mastectomy, already outlined above. The word play in the title 'Cutting Deadly Odds' literalizes the cultural fear of both cancer and mutilation of the feminine form. 'The Breast Cancer Family' story functions within the same rhetorical paradigm, substituting phrases like 'chopped off' and 'cut off' instead of using the term 'mastectomy':

If there have been no medical advances then I'll have them chopped off. (*The Observer*, 30 June 1996)

... the body has to be attacked to be treated. We cut off bits of ourselves in order to save the rest. (*The Observer*, 30 June 1996)

The public sense of horror, of mastectomy itself, but compounded by the notion of removing the healthy breasts of (young) women, governs the language featured in these narratives, and is emphasized through the use of hyperbole and dramatic overstatement:

These sisters are healthy yet they each want both breasts removed. (*Scottish Mirror*, 29 May 1996)

She wasn't feeling ill and there was no physical sign she had cancer. But Wendy Watson decided to have both breasts removed – as soon as possible. (*Scottish Mirror*, 14 February 1996)

I'm young and healthy and I'm going to have my breasts cut off. (*The Observer*, 30 June 1996)

Continuing in this vein and anticipating cultural understandings of mastectomy, individual decisions to undertake prophylactic surgery are foregrounded as 'extreme' (*Scottish Mirror,* 14 February and 9 October 1996) 'a drastic step' (*Scottish Mirror,* 29 May 1996), and the result of 'panicky' or 'irrational' decisions (*Scottish Mirror,* 29 May 1996). The rationale of decisions made by women with a high inherited risk is defended by couching cancer risk in terms of inevitability by emphasizing the 'deadliness' of 'the gene'. Correspondingly, the breast is detached, sometimes quite literally, from its feminine and sexual associations. One subject is cited as follows: 'for most women, breasts are about being a woman, being sexy, being a mother. But for me they were about fear, death' (The Breast Cancer Family, *The Observer,* 30 June 1996).

None the less, most accounts frame the impact of breast loss in terms of sexual attraction. All the articles listed above discuss the impact of mastectomy in terms of sexual practice and relationship status. In 'Cutting Deadly Odds', Andrea, a married mother of two, opts to have all the breast tissue and nipples removed. Her unmarried sister decides to keep her nipples and some of the tissue. She is quoted as follows: 'I don't think I could have coped with losing my breasts altogether ... I'm still single and it might put some men off' (*Scottish Mirror,* 29 May 1996). Sometimes partners of subjects speak for them. In '17 in my Family ... ' Jayne's husband says: 'Nothing has changed ... We have a good sex life, even though Jayne no longer has any feeling in her breasts' (*Scottish Mirror,* 9 October 1996).

Only one of the articles above references the effects of mastectomy in terms of its impact outside of sexuality and maternity. In '17 in my Family ...' Jayne says: 'There is nothing I can't do. I still do aerobics and swim' (*ibid.*). This was the sole reference to any aspect of the impact of mastectomy on anything other than sex and attraction.

While traditional ideas of femininity are threatened by both preventative and therapeutic breast surgery, narrative allusions to vanity are situated in a moral framework and posited implicitly as irresponsible and irrational. In 'The Breast Cancer Family' prophylactic mastectomy is situated as optional for women at risk. However, the notion of choice is undermined by being juxtaposed against a moral fable. A consultant geneticist is cited saying: 'I would never tell anyone what to do ... Some women would never choose to have a radical mastectomy when they are perfectly healthy'. His statement is followed by an account of a woman *already diagnosed with a cancerous tumour* (as opposed to the healthy women with a high inherited risk who are the subject of the article):

> Stella was engaged to be married when she discovered a cancerous tumour in her breast. She took medical advice and also spent many hours with counsellors in the breast clinic. And then she decided, to their concealed distress, not to do anything, at least until after the wedding. She wanted to be whole on her big day. She married and was beautiful; the tumour spread; later she had a mastectomy; her husband left her; she is now undergoing chemotherapy. Her image of herself was so destroyed by the idea of cutting off her breast that she preferred to risk her life. She lies in a hospital bed, and the wedding dress hangs in her cupboard. (*The Observer*, 30 June 1996)

This contrasts starkly with the testimonies of two other women, each with the gene (but not cancer) in the same article:

> ... I'm familiar with cancer, so I'm not so scared of it. I have a cancer gene and I reckon I have about eight years, till I'm 30, to decide what to do. If there have been no medical advances, then I'll have them chopped off. It's not ideal ... but my partner doesn't mind and now I know he loves me for myself and not my tits.

> I'm not brave, I just didn't want to die. I have a lovely daughter, and I breast-fed her, and my sex life is still excellent, and my husband has had no problems.

The rhetorical purpose of the comparison is obviously to support the pro-mastectomy choices made by high-risk women. However, the contrast unfairly undermines the choices and fears of women facing difficult preventative or therapeutic decisions, especially given the emphasis on the cosmetic impact of breast cancer in media reporting.

In stories about prophylactic mastectomy, the maternal status of subjects is often emphasized. This was not restricted to this sub-genre of breast cancer reporting. In fact, the most conspicuous figure in breast cancer narratives was that of the mother. In the above sample, mothers were central as narrative subjects – more than 70 per cent of personal accounts of 'ordinary' women included reference to parental status and more than 20 per cent of the personal accounts focused on motherhood as the main story. In breast cancer narratives, mother-hood is couched in terms of martyrdom and self-sacrifice. Through this heavy emphasis, breast cancer narratives situate the illness in a particular trajectory of life-events whereby feminine worth is preordained and what is at stake fits neatly into a moral order within which the central character is unquestioningly heroic. Where understandings of femininity based on bodily constructions are challenged by breast disease, moral conceptions are emphasized. Cultural constructions of maternity idealize mothers who privilege the well-being of others over themselves.

In stories about prophylactic surgery and inherited risk, subjects were often positioned as mothers and their choice framed as sacrifice. Mothers with a high inherited risk sacrifice their breasts for their children, and agonize about their 'flawed' genes affecting children and grandchildren:

Jayne makes agonising sacrifice so she can see her boys grow up (*Scottish Mirror*, 9 October 1996)

... after Andrea's children were born she felt she couldn't ignore the problem any longer ... 'I'd look at my children and think: I can't bear the thought of a third generation of our family growing up without a mother'. (*Scottish Mirror*, 29 May 1996)

I may not have a daughter to worry about, but I still think about what will happen if my sons have daughters ... (*Scottish Mirror*, 9 October 1996)

It's hard for me, for my husband, and I'm very aware of my three daughters. Obviously they've probably got the gene too, but they're still very little ... (*The Observer*, 30 June 1996)

This theme was definitively elaborated in another sub-genre of breast cancer reporting. Maternal-centred narratives were dominated by tragedies and triumphs which focused on (young) mothers who risked their lives for their unborn children. Over half of the personal accounts about mothers centred on women who risked or sacrificed their lives for their unborn children. This was the case in both broadsheet and tabloid press.

This sub-genre defines its heroine according to her (intended) sacrifice. The woman who terminates a pregnancy is a morally dubious figure in popular culture. She is potentially redeemable, hypothetically speaking, if abortion is motivated by the risk to her life. None the less, there was not a single account focused on a woman who chose abortion and a full course of treatment. The woman who gives her life, or is willing to give her life, for her (unborn) child offers the ultimate sacrifice. (Interestingly, none of the subjects had any other children. All were giving birth for the first time, so the question of sacrifice was uncomplicated by other maternal obligations. This simplified the motivation underlying the narratives.) In this sub-genre, the loss of a breast takes a narratorial back seat, and the loss of the maternal life, where it occurs, is particularly poignant.

In all of the mother-centred stories women were depicted using metaphors of sainthood and martyrdom – they were archetypically self-sacrificing women. The following headlines exemplify this:

Mummy Gave Her Life So I Can Live (*The Sun,* 17 February 1995)

I Must Choose – My Life or My Babies (*Scottish Mirror,* 13 March 1996)

Baby Joy for Cancer Mum (*The Sun,* 2 April 1997)

Mother Turns down Cancer Treatment to Save Unborn Baby (*The Times,* 20 March 1996)

The theme of self-negation was most prominent in the article head-lined 'Mummy Gave Her Life so I Can Live' (*The Sun,* 17 February 1995). This was a story about a mother who refused treatment because it would damage her unborn child. Melodramatic pathos is intensified in this article through the headline assuming the narrative position of the child, and through the opening paragraph which introduces a dialogue between the child and father at the graveside of the dead mother. The woman is characterized as both martyr and hero in a way typical of cancer narratives (Stacey 1997) and the child is situated as a legacy of the mother's sacrifice: 'Marina refused full treatment for breast cancer, knowing her baby would stand a better chance, although it would make her hopes of survival slim'. Her husband is quoted saying: 'She was a marvel. She would come back tired and list-less and feeling sick from the treatment but she never complained and carried on, like the fighter she was.'

Similar rhetorical strategies appeared in other articles in which preg-nant women delayed chemotherapy treatment. In 'I Must Choose – My Life or My Babies' (*Scottish Mirror,* 13 March 1996), Alex discovered she had breast cancer on the same day she was told she was pregnant with twins:

I found myself facing the biggest decision of my life. I could have chemotherapy and, because we'd caught the cancer early, probably survive. But I'd have to terminate the pregnancy and lose my precious babies. Or I could put my life on the line by letting the babies grow inside me while the cancer grew too. I would have to have a mastectomy followed by a Caesarean – by which time the cancer could have riddled my body ... [She decided:] I would have my babies. Their lives were more important than mine.

The case of Sonya Short followed a similar trajectory. Published in *The Times* and *The Independent*, both papers followed up on the story when Short was cured of cancer in April (e.g. 'Mother Who Delayed Cure in Clear', *The Times* 8 April 1996). She was valorized for her decision to sacrifice her breast rather than have chemotherapy which would have threatened the life of her then unborn son. Similarly, the story of Polly Carnegie was covered in *The Times* and *The Sun* after Carnegie, advised to terminate her pregnancy, instead delayed her chemotherapy treatment until after the baby was fully formed. The prevalence of mother/tragedy/triumph narratives in breast cancer stories, then, testifies to the centrality of the archetypal maternal (i.e. self-sacrificing) heroine.

Stories about breast cancer are governed by preconceptions of the 'horror' of removing healthy breasts, and the resultant impact on conceptions of femininity as sexuality and maternity. Frequently and implicitly, stories subscribe to a rigid and limited definition of femininity, bodily based and youth-centred, threatened by notions of mutilation, reinforced by maternal sacrifice and rescued by reconstruction and recovered (hetero)sexual attraction.

'Alternative' Visual and Narrative Representations of Breast Cancer

The images and stories discussed so far conceptualize breast cancer within limited definitions of femininity. The paradigms of representation discussed detract from the many ways in which women might experience breast cancer and limit the positions from which readers might identify. Breast cancer is, as one breast care nurse pointed out during the course of this study, not one disease but many. As such, it is experienced physiologically in very different ways by the women afflicted. Add to this the complex variables through which women experience their bodies and femininity – such as age, class, race and sexuality – and the representations discussed earlier might appear somewhat reductive, in so far as their frequency and framing assumes a norm to the exclusion of alternative accounts.

Breast cancer narratives published outside the popular media testify to this. Eve Kozofsky Sedgewick, in her book *Tendencies*, criticizes the notion that breasts are inherently central to every woman's sense of gender identity and integrity:

> This did not happen to be my situation: as a person who has been non-procreative by choice, and whose sense of femininity, whatever it many consist in, has never been routed through a pretty appearance in the imagined view of heterosexual men – as a woman moreover whose breast eroticism wasn't strong – I was someone to whom these mammary globes, though pleasing in myself and in others who sported them, were nonetheless relatively peripheral to the complex places where sexuality and gender identity really happen. (1993: 262)

Sedgewick found that chemotherapy and its associated hair loss were far more of a challenge to her gendered identity than breast removal.

Audre Lorde, in a well-known passage from *The Cancer Journals*, describes an incident which impresses the specificity of her experience as a black lesbian sufferer of breast cancer. She recounts how, while in the hospital, a volunteer from Reach for Recovery visited bringing a pale pink prosthesis, ostensibly to aid her recovery:

> Her message was, you are just as good as you were before because you can look exactly the same ... nobody'll ever know the difference ... 'Look at me,' she said ... standing before me in a tight blue sweater ... 'Now can you tell which is which?' I admitted that I could not. In her tight foundation garment and stiff, uplifting bra, both breasts looked equally unreal to me. But then I've always been a connoisseur of women's breasts, and never overly fond of stiff uplifts. I looked away, thinking, 'I wonder if there are any black lesbian feminists in Reach for Recovery?' (Lorde 1988: 31)

Occasionally, alternative, critical or self-reflexive representations find their way into mainstream media accounts. Perhaps the most obvious example of this is an American instance: a 1993 *New York*

Times cover featured model Matuschka, dressed in a garment cut diagonally to reveal her mastectomized chest while covering the remaining breast. The picture was lit like a fashion photograph to highlight her scar, and the image was titled 'Beauty out of Damage'. The feature elicited some very negative reactions: embarrassment, disgust and shame – particularly from survivors. Some felt it had invaded their privacy, that people would know what they really looked like (Matuschka 1993). Other responses however, were quite positive. Matuschka argued:

> If we keep quiet about what breast cancer does to women's bodies, if we refuse to accept women's bodies in whatever condition they are in, we are doing a disservice to womankind ... I hope that my image will convey the idea that a woman with one breast or no breasts (*sic*) is entitled to be looked at and approved of. (*ibid.*)

Despite the enormous publicity generated by Matuschka's image, it remains a rare instance for which there is no British equivalent. In a recent news feature 'Scars and Bras' (*The Guardian,* 28 September 1998) breast cancer survivor Julia Darling draws attention to this:

> I felt I didn't have a model, or a way of imagining my body after the operation. There were Jo Spence's important but angry self-portraits and the emotionless images in medical books but that was it. There are still pitifully few images of women who choose not to wear prostheses. You can't buy clothes to fit one-breasted women at any High Street shop. If one in twelve women have had breast cancer, that's an awful lot of women whose condition is not reflected in the wider world.

Darling describes how her choice of a double mastectomy (her cancer had only affected one breast) was not allowed by her hospital, which would not sanction the removal of healthy breasts. However, it did offer the more expensive, and, it must be argued, more culturally acceptable, option of reconstructive surgery. In 'Bras and Scars' she states:

> There is something creepy about the premise that you have to have two breasts to be complete and the idea that the experience of breast cancer can be covered up, as if it never happened, and women can be remade so they are almost as good as new ... Every

time I see someone who flaunts the fact that she has one lump, not two, I feel like cheering.

Darling eventually persuaded her doctor to remove the remaining breast and described the impact of this as follows: 'These days I can wear a vest and feel agile and unhampered. Swimming is easier; so is jumping up and down. I know I have reclaimed myself.'

The final part of this chapter explores two alternative media accounts of breast cancer, published in broadsheet newspapers: Ruth Picardie's column in *The Observer*, 'Before I Say Goodbye' (published in full, 19 October 1997); and Kathy Acker's feature article in *The Guardian*, 'The Gift of Disease' (18 January 1997). The term 'alternative' in this instance refers to divergences from the discourses discussed earlier, which construct the images and experiences of breast cancer within the confines of acceptable definitions of femininity and illness. While Picardie and Acker speak from very different perspectives, both accounts are self-consciously distanced from many of the dominant discourses for representing breast cancer and each generated a large public response which focused on the alternative emphases of Acker's and Picardie's experiences. However, they are not necessarily, or definitively, transgressive or radical accounts.

Acker's representations of her experience of cancer and her post-mastectomy body is facilitated by her public persona as a literary celebrity and by her well-known avantgarde body politics. Renowned for her tattooing and multiple body piercing as much as her outrageous writing and performance art, obituaries following her recent death bore titles like 'Power Punk and Porn' (*The Guardian*, 1 December 1997, p. 13) and 'A Pirate, A Pioneer; a Punk Princess' (*The Independent*, 2 December 1997 p. 19). Since Acker was known for challenging accepted notions of gender and sexuality, it is not surprising that her experience does not comply with the more generic accounts of breast cancer.

In 'The Gift of Disease', Acker's experience is recounted as a blow-by-blow description of the experience of surgery, including dialogue that is organized and presented like a script. Acker refers to her body abstractly as 'diseased meat', and to her struggle as being against mere materiality. She politicizes her experience by outlining her reasons for abandoning conventional medicine for alternative healing, and situates cancer treatment in a market economy.

Acker opted for a double mastectomy, though her cancer only affected one breast. Her decision is framed by the financial constraints limiting and defining the very notion of 'choice':

> Since I didn't have medical insurance, I would have to pay for everything out of my pocket. Radiation on its own costs $20,000; a single mastectomy costs approximately $4,000. Of course, there would be extra expenses. I chose a double mastectomy, for I did not want to have only one breast. The price was $7,000, I could afford to pay for that. Breast reconstruction, in which I had no interest, begins at $20,000. Chemotherapy, likewise, begins at $20,000. (1997: 14)

(While Acker underwent treatment in the US, similar constraints are experienced by women seeking treatment in the UK as Julia Darling's account mentioned above illustrates.)

None the less, Acker situates her choice as directed by a desire for bodily symmetry, though not a conventionally defined curvaceous feminine form. 'The Gift of Disease' is accompanied by photographs of Acker which do not attempt to hide the evidence of her mastectomy. Generically, the photographs avoid the categories within which survivors are usually imaged (i.e. in familial contexts, or smiling and showing no evidence of breast surgery, or shot from the neck down). Acker is framed using the conventions of fashion photography. In one image, which featured on the cover of *The Guardian's* 'Weekend' magazine, she is pictured wearing a low cut feathery fake-fur wrap. She reveals a large expanse of bare flat chest, and leans forward to highlight this. In another picture, which took up a whole page, Acker wears a tight fitting leopard print shirt, open almost to her midriff. Evidence of her double mastectomy is clearly depicted in the absence of any kind of cleavage and the image is lit to draw attention to this. In her clothing and stance then, Acker plays with the props which define conventions of femininity and sexuality.

Ruth Picardie's account described breast cancer from a very different perspective from that of Kathy Acker. Perhaps the first thing that defines its specificity in relation to many of the accounts discussed so far is that Picardie's experience didn't involve breast loss. In a contribution to a feature about breasts published by *The Independent*, she described how this shaped her experience of cancer:

> For me, breast cancer is not really about breasts, it's about life and death. You've got a life-threatening illness, you've got to have horrible treatment, but the breasts are irrelevant. Breast cancer is a

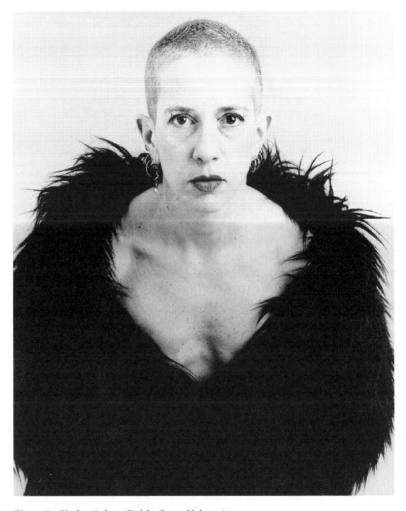

Figure 1   Kathy Acker (*Del LaGrace Volcano*).

very counter-intuitive illness because it doesn't make you feel ill. You feel fine. Then you have chemotherapy, your hair falls out and you think, 'Maybe I am going to die'. ('Me and my Breasts', 15 February 1997, p. 14)

Picardie's account of breast cancer has generated considerable interest and concern in the UK. Titled 'Before I Say Goodbye', it was first published as a regular column over three months and in seven separate articles, the last of which was published just prior to her death. The episodic structure of the account lends it particular poignancy – the series began before she knew her cancer was terminal and the final instalment was completed by her sister (who is Features Editor for the 'Life' section of *The Observer*, where the account was first published). In many ways the story contained the raw material defining the tragic cancer narratives discussed earlier – Picardie was a young, attractive, married mother. Her column was accompanied by colour photographs of her and her children and she frequently wrote about them. This perhaps accounts for the broad appeal of the story. In addition to its publication as a series in *The Observer*, it was reproduced in full by the paper following her death, and was also reproduced as a series for a national tabloid, *The Express*. Later, Picardie's story along with letters, e-mails and contributions from her husband and family, was published as a book (*Before I Say Goodbye*, Penguin, 1998).

Her narrative may be described as 'alternative' because of its self-reflexivity. As well as describing an experience which is not 'breast-centred' in the way that various accounts of lumpectomy and mastectomy customarily are, 'Before I Say Goodbye' is marked by the writer's awareness of the narrative conventions inherent in describing illness and femininity. Picardie's relative degree of editorial control perhaps had a hand in her self-conscious subversion of the kinds of discourses discussed earlier. Her account is defined by its humour and bitter irony, as she tells of plotting to get subsidized cleaning, of comfort eating and unsuccessful attempts at alternative therapies.

In 'Before I Say Goodbye' Picardie refused the traditional stance of the stoic fighter and selfless martyr which defines the mother/fighter sub-genre discussed earlier. In one column she states:

> ... having a terminal illness is supposed to make you extremely wise and evolved, turning you into the kind of person who thinks: 'What is being 11 stone compared with the joy of seeing my children run through a flowery meadow as if in a junior Timotei ad? (1998: 17)

Instead, Picardie detailed her resentment at how unglamorous breast cancer felt as an illness. Ironically, while she stated that 'breast cancer = old ladies in wigs' (p. 17), this is precisely the image of breast cancer that media accounts downplay. Picardie's discussion of cancer included direct references to conceptions usually tucked away behind metaphors and euphemisms. For example, in one column, Picardie describes her cancer as being like a pregnancy. This analogy is common in discourses about cancer, as Jackie Stacey points out in *Teratologies*, paralleling the monstrous 'hijacked' body harbouring cancer with the grotesqueness of femininity and fertility (1997: 87–91). Picardie refers directly to this, though with a degree of humour, even while alluding to the taboo of death (and her own imminent death, at that):

> Sadly, being diagnosed with cancer seems to have arrested my capacity for high-powered psychological evolution. For – a shocking 10 months since Diagnosis Day – I have become convinced that I am, in fact, pregnant. Which, on the face of it, is down there in the kindergarten of denial ... However, I only need to refer you to one of the pregnancy manuals dusting up my shelves: the vomiting, the weird stuff growing inside you, the endless waiting for the big day ... (1998: 21)

Picardie's experience of her femininity was challenged by chemotherapy with its associated pubic hair loss and weight gain. (While it might be argued that this was because she didn't experience breast loss, Eve Kozofsky Sedgewick, in *Tendencies*, also details how hair loss played havoc with her gender identity, even though she had undergone mastectomy (1993: 12–15, 263).) Picardie bemoans the irony of how chemotherapy made her look healthy, or simply fat, instead of causing her to fade away to the image of translucent tuberculine beauty associated with glamorous illness, and discussed by Susan Sontag in *Illness As Metaphor* (1978). She describes the pleasures of 'retail therapy' even while shopping for a post-chemotherapy body, in rather grotesque, but none the less humorous, terms:

> My symptoms are a slightly swollen brain, but I'm hoping today's lunch (smoked salmon bagels, crisps, extra French dressing) will have a positive effect. The other problem – my enlarged liver – I believe has been solved by my later splurge at the Whistles sale (blue skirt, lilac shirt). Even if the dread organ does not shrink, the clever bias cutting hides most of the lumps. (1998: 21)

While humorously detailing her thwarted expectations, Picardie often soberly acknowledged the reality of cancer. After detailing her frustration at her body's defiance of her expectations of weight loss and ethereal femininity, she finished one column stating: 'someone at my support group recently lost a lot of weight. On Monday night, she died. I'm glad I look well, after all' (*ibid.* 18). Picardie's experience of breast cancer, then, is obviously shaped by factors other than gender, such as class – her therapeutic indulgences would not be available to a working-class woman in a similar situation. Her story does not, however, assume any universally feminine representation of the experience of breast cancer. Moreover, the way in which the illness impacts in terms of her gender identity is fragmented and diffuse, defying the rigidity of those categories which shape the experience of breast cancer in terms of sexual and maternal femininity.

In conclusion, breast cancer is made newsworthy in most media reporting by focusing on the experiences of young and either maternal or sexual female bodies. This is influenced by perceptions of femininity which focus on the breast as an icon of feminine worth. This is not necessarily the way in which women understand or experience breast cancer. For example, one study (Luker et al. 1996) found that information about sexual attractiveness was ranked least important by women following diagnoses and treatment for breast cancer. The press focus on the breast obscures other dimensions of the experience and polices how women should experience their bodies (for example, assuming that mastectomies must be hidden and reconstruction is mandatory). It also ignores all the other bodily effects of cancer and its treatment; from swollen organs to the loss of hair. Such bodily effects may be a very important part of the experience.

Notes

1 This has involved interviews with specialist medical and science correspondents, focus group discussions with women and health professionals and analysis of three years' press coverage of breast cancer.
2 The following chart illustrates the increasing publicity of breast cancer. It is based on a CD-Rom search of three UK national broadsheet newspapers and their sister Sunday papers. (*The Times* and *The Sunday Times* could only be searched for 1996 and 1997 as previous years were not available on CD-Rom.) The search was for all articles citing the term 'breast cancer' in text. The graph illustrates a steady increase in media coverage of breast cancer in national broadsheet newspapers.

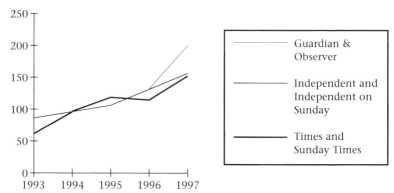

Articles including the term 'breast cancer' in text in three major broadsheets, 1993–1997

3   In our study, breast cancer was by far the most commonly mentioned cancer in broadsheet newspapers, both in headlines and in text, from 1995 to 1997. It was headlined four times as often as any other cancer, and referenced in text almost twice as often as other cancers.

Cancers in the News: The Guardian and Observer, The Independent and Independent on Sunday, The Times and Sunday Times, 1995–1997

	Headlines	References in Text
Breast cancer	133	1243
Lung cancer	18	750
Prostate cancer	31	466
Skin cancer	26	362
Testicular cancer	1	154
Liver cancer	1	108
Ovarian cancer	4	128
Bowel cancer	9	103
Stomach cancer	0	154
Cervical cancer	15	193
Colon cancer	0	76

4   These figures exclude celebrity subjects because their newsworthiness can be attributed to celebrity status rather than breast cancer as such. When celebrities are included, the age breakdown of subjects is as follows: 38 per cent of subjects were 35 years or under; 39 per cent were aged 36–49; 22 per cent were aged 50–65; 1 per cent were over 65 years of age.

5   Except for women with the breast cancer gene, mammography as a prophylactic technique is less applicable to younger women, first, because they are
less at risk, and second, because younger breasts are denser and less likely to
show pre-cancerous lumps.
6   We were only able to index a full sample of images from the tabloid press
as broadsheet dailies and Sundays newspapers were obtained through CD-
Rom searches.

Acknowledgement

This chapter derives from a project entitled 'The Role of the Media in Public
and Professional Understanding of Breast Cancer', funded by the NHS
Executive Research and Development Programme from January 1996 to
December 1997. The grant holders were Jenny Kitzinger and Greg Philo.

References
Brooks, L. 'The Mark of a Woman'. *The Guardian Weekend* (14 November 1998)
pp. 26–32.
Cartwright, L. 'Community and the Public Body in Breast Cancer Activism'.
Cultural Studies 12 (2) (1998) pp. 117–38.
CRC Institute for Cancer Studies at the University of Birmingham. (1997)
Cancerhelp UK Breast Cancer Overview (1997). http://medweb.bhm.cncer-
help /public /specific/ breast/index.html
Henderson, L. 'Making Health News! Media Values, Source Strategies and
Breast Cancer Research'. Paper presented BSA Medical Sociology Conference,
York, September 1997.
Lorde, A. *The Cancer Journals. In The Audre Lorde Compendium: Essays, Speeches
and Journals* (London: HarperCollins 1988).
Luker, K.A., K. Beaver, S.J. Leinster and R. Glynn Owens. 'Information Needs
and Sources of Information For Women With Breast Cancer: A Follow-Up
Study'. *Journal of Advanced Nursing* 23 (1996) pp. 487–95.
Matuschka. Matuschka explains the NYT photo in her article 'Why I Did It'
(originally appeared in *Glamour Magazine*, November 1993). http://
www.itp.tsoa.nyu.edu/~student/pincushion/FORUMHTML/why/html
Sedgwick, E.K. *Tendencies* (Durham, NC: Duke University Press 1993).
Solomon, A. 'The Politics of Breast Cancer'. *Camera Obscura: A Journal of
Feminism and Film Theory*, 28 (1995) pp. 157–77.
Sontag, S. *Illness as Metaphor* (New York: Farrer, Strauss & Giroux 1978).
Stacey, J. *Teratologies* (London: Routledge 1997).
Voda, A. M. Review of *The Meaning of Menopause: Historical, Medical & Clinical
Perspectives*, ed. Ruth Formanek (Hillsdale NJ: Analytic Press, 1990) in *Signs*,
18 (1993) pp. 447–51.
Yalom, M. *A History of the Breast* (London & New York, HarperCollins 1997).

News Sources (By Title)

An Ad Too Far from the Tofu and Muesli Merchants, by Colin Blackstock,
Independent on Sunday (19 October 1997) p. 3.

Baby Joy For Cancer Mum, by Dr Rosemary, *The Sun* (2 April 1997) p. 4.

Beast in the Breast, by Judy Sadgrove, *The Guardian* (29 October 1996) p. 10.

Beauty and the Breast, by John Illman, *The Guardian* (3 October 1995) p. 14.

Before I Say Goodbye, by Ruth Picardie. (7 parts, published in full). *The Observer (Life Section)* (19 October 1997) pp. 14–24.

The Breast Cancer Family, by Nicci Gerrard, *The Observer* (30 June 1996) p. 9.

Breast Op Doc Made Me a Freak, *Daily Record* (10 April 1997) p. 1, 2–3.

The Breast Option, *The Sun* (10 January 1996) pp. 6–7.

Cancer Victim's Baby, *The Independent* (20 March 1996) p. 2.

Cutting Deadly Odds, by Catriona Wrottesley *Scottish Mirror* (29 May 1996) pp. 6–7.

Doctor at Large: Keeping Abreast of the Facts, by Luisa Dillner, *The Guardian* (14 January 1997) p. 18.

The Gift of Disease, by Kathy Acker, *The Guardian, Weekend Supplement* (18 January 1997) pp. 14–21.

Girls Go to War, by Helen Weathers, *Scottish Mirror* (4 April 1996) p. 6.

I Must Choose – My Life or My Babies, by Sarah Hey *Scottish Mirror* (13 March 1996) pp. 2–3.

I Partied My Way through Chemo, by Vicky Grimshaw *The Sun* (8 October 1997) pp. 4–5.

I Thought Men Didn't Get Breast Cancer, *Daily Mirror* (20 March 1995) pp. 28–9.

If Cancer Runs in a Family, by Dr Trisha Greenhalgh *The Times* (11 April 1995) p. 14.

It's a Bra-illiant Idea, *Scottish Mirror* (11 June 1997) p. 8.

Keeping abreast of Breast Cancer, *The Guardian* (9 September 1995) p. 26.

Knockers Slate New Breast Ads, by Colin Guthrie MD. *The Sun* (27 December 1997) p. 38.

Mother Turns down Cancer Treatment to Save Unborn Baby, *The Times* (20 March 1996).

Mother Who Delayed Cure in Clear, *The Times* (8 April 1996).

Mummy Gave Her Life So I Can Live, by Vicky Grimshaw, *The Sun* (17 February 1995) pp. 38–9.

9 of My Family Got Cancer so I Had My Breasts Removed In Case I Was The Next, by Catriona Wrottesley, *Scottish Mirror* (14 February 1996) pp. 7–8.

Scars and Bras, by Hilary Bower, *The Guardian* (28 September 1998) pp. 6–7.

17 in My Family Have Died from Breast Cancer, by Emma Creamer, *Scottish Mirror* (9 October 1996) pp. 10–11.

The Unbearable Naked Truth, by Clare Dyer, *The Guardian* (16 April 1996) p. 13.

Women at Risk of Cancer Agonise over Mastectomy, by Jeremy Laurance, *The Times* (26 February 1996) p. 14.

3
Racing for the Cure, Walking Women and Toxic Touring: Mapping Cultures of Action within the Bay Area Terrain of Breast Cancer

Maren Klawiter

> The main function of public spaces is that of rendering visible and collective the questions raised by movements.
> Alberto Melucci (1994: 189)

Beginning in the second half of the 1980s and gathering momentum in the 1990s, new forms of cancer organizing, activism and community began to proliferate across the United States. Within a decade, a wide range of networks, projects, organizations, foundations, coalitions and public events arose that expanded and challenged the way that cancer, and breast cancer in particular, had been publicly framed and institutionally managed. Although this was not the first time that cancer had entered the 'universe of discourse' (Bourdieu, 1977) and been transformed into an object of political debate and public scrutiny, the cultures of action that mushroomed in the late 1980s and expanded during the 1990s introduced onto the historical landscape a new set of social actors, cultural practices and political logics. Unlike earlier historical moments in which cancer as a broad category had occupied centre stage, this time it was breast cancer that moved to the centre, and it was breast cancer survivors and activists who moved it there.[1]

In 1993 the breast cancer movement – or at least one slice of it – arrived on the cover of the *New York Times Magazine (NYT)*. The cover of the 15 August issue featured a self-portrait of the breast cancer activist and artist Matuschka with one half of the bodice of her elegant white dress cut away to expose a mastectomy scar where her right breast had been. The cover story, entitled '"You Can't Look Away Anymore": The Anguished Politics of Breast Cancer' (Ferraro 1993), focused on the rapid rise and remarkable success of the National Breast Cancer Coalition (NBCC), a Washington DC-based feminist lobbying organization founded in 1991. In the *NYT* article, the agenda of the breast cancer movement – with NBCC as its symbolic representative – was defined as raising public awareness, increasing the influence of breast cancer survivors and expanding the federal budget for breast cancer research.

This issue of the *NYT* received four times the usual volume of letters to the editor (Batt 1994). Interestingly enough, it seemed to be the cover photo, as much as the content of the article, that inspired the flurry of letter-writing. The image of Matuschka – the public display of her one-breasted body – had struck a powerful chord. The range and intensity of responses to this article and to Matuschka's style of embodied activism suggested that widespread support for the general goals of the NBCC might be concealing important differences within the broader terrain of breast cancer activism.

In 1994, I began studying how breast cancer was being publicly reshaped and politicized in the San Francisco Bay Area. But instead of studying the dynamics of change and challenge within national lobbying campaigns, I chose to explore the local terrain of action. In the Bay Area I discovered a multifaceted movement that was in full swing. However, within this arena the National Breast Cancer Coalition – the force consistently defined by itself and the media as *the* breast cancer movement – was organizationally absent and discursively marginal. What I discovered instead was a dynamic, diverse and expanding field of local grassroots activity.

I use the differences within the Bay Area terrain of breast cancer activism to contribute to scholarship on the breast cancer movement and to theorize at the juncture of culture and social movements. Through participant observation[2] I develop thick descriptions, or representations, of three social movement spectacles and analyse them as loci for the production, performance and circulation of new social actors, cultural practices and political logics – or what I conceptualize as three different *cultures of action*. I use the concept *culture of action* to emphasize that culture within social movements is publicly produced and performed through an assembly of practices that are enacted, enunciated, emoted and embodied.

By paying attention to the different ways in which breast cancer is enacted, enunciated, emoted and embodied, I disaggregate the Bay

Area field of breast cancer activism into three different cultures of action. The first, represented by Race for the Cure®, draws upon biomedicine and private industry, and emphasizes individual agency, honour and survival. It connects breast cancer to the display of normative femininities, mobilizes hope and faith in science and medicine, and promotes biomedical research and early detection. The second, represented by the Women & Cancer Walk, draws upon multicultural feminism, the women's health movement and AIDS activism. It connects breast cancer to other women's cancers, challenges the emphasis on survival and the hegemonic display of heteronormative femininities, emphasizes the effects of institutionalized inequalities, mobilizes anger against the institutions of biomedicine, and promotes social services and treatment activism. The third, represented by the Toxic Tour of the Cancer Industry, draws upon the feminist cancer and environmental justice movements and broadens the focus to include all cancers and environmentally related illnesses. It represents breast cancer as both the product and source of profits of a global cancer industry, mobilizes outrage against corporate malfeasance and environmental racism and replaces the emphasis on biomedical research and early detection with demands for corporate regulation and cancer prevention.

Feminist Approaches to Breast Cancer Activism

Only a small number of scholars have studied the breast cancer movement and they have analysed it by posing questions that engage most directly with the sociology of emotions (Montini 1996), the sociology of gender (Taylor and Van Willigen 1996) and the sociology of science (Anglin 1997). The first study, conducted by Montini (1996), examined the wave of breast cancer informed-consent legislation that swept across the United States during the 1980s. In 22 states, legislation was introduced that required physicians to inform their patients of treatment options and obtain their consent before proceeding. In each state, the legislative effort constituted a small-scale phenomenon that involved only a handful of former breast cancer patients who operated in isolation from broader social movement communities. Montini showed how these breast cancer activists strategically drew upon conservative norms of heterofemininity in their media presentations and public testimonies. As part of their script, they positioned themselves as the victims of callous surgeons and in need of state protections; they avoided the public display of anger – although they expressed it in private – and they displayed instead the gender-norma-tive emotions of fear and grief. Montini argued that, in so doing, they reproduced conservative norms of femininity and extended them to a new political subject: the breast cancer patient. Although informed consent legislation was successfully passed in 16 states by 1989, breast cancer activism in the 1980s remained narrowly focused on specific legislative goals, and was sustained by a handful of individuals rather than by broader social movements.

Taylor and Van Willigen (1996) published the first sociological study of the breast cancer movement of the 1990s. Drawing upon Taylor's research on the postpartum depression movement and Van Willigen's research on the breast cancer movement, they traced the genealogies of both mobilizations to the cultural and political reper-toires of self-help groups and to the larger phenomenon of women's self-help movements of the past two decades. Taylor and Van Willigen argued that women's self-help movements had, in recent years, been maligned as 'apolitical' by one strand of scholars within feminism, and dismissed as 'not a social movement' by many scholars within sociology. They used their research to construct a counternarrative, demonstrating that breast cancer activists challenged the gender order by identifying themselves as 'breast cancer survivors', refusing to wear breast prostheses, demanding access to medical information, chal-lenging the boundaries of allopathic medicine, and creating new social networks and supportive spaces. Taylor and Van Willigen thus argued that the breast cancer and postpartum depression movements – and women's self-help movements in general – challenged the insti-tution of gender along three different dimensions: as a process; a hierarchy; and a structure – a conceptualization of gender as an insti-tution based on the work of Judith Lorber (1994).

Finally, Anglin (1997) used her ethnography of a breast cancer orga-nization to explore the ways in which treatment activism during the early 1990s challenged the power relations embedded within science and medicine. Whereas Montini's activists in the 1980s were posi-tioned as individual, victimized patients operating outside the context of a broader social movement, Anglin's breast cancer activists belonged to just such a movement, made up of more than 300 breast cancer organizations united in their demands for more research and better treatment alternatives. Anglin drew primarily upon literature within the sociology of knowledge and science to analyse the chal-lenges posed by breast cancer treatment activism to structures of power within science and medicine. At the same time, she used her case-study to argue that treatment activism was being narrowly defined from the privileged social, medical and cultural location of a predominantly white and middle-class constituency.

My analysis touches upon themes that have been identified and explored by these scholars. For example, I analyse the ways in which gender styles and emotions are publicly mobilized and enacted (Montini 1996; Taylor and Van Willigen 1996). I also explore some of the ways that breast cancer activism discursively engages the authority and priorities of science and medicine (Anglin 1997; Taylor and Van Willigen 1996). And I pay attention to the workings of power and to questions of position, representation and exclusion (Anglin 1997). But instead of identifying commonalities and developing an analysis of the breast cancer movement as a whole,[3] I seek to identify, disentangle and analyse different strands of activism around breast cancer. Thus, instead of situating my analysis within the sociology of emotions (Montini 1996), gender and social movements (Taylor and Van Willigen 1996) or the sociology of science (Anglin 1997), I approach the local terrain of breast cancer activism from an angle of vision opened up by recent developments at the juncture of culture and social movements.

Theorizing at the Juncture of Culture and Social Movements

This chapter draws upon and contributes to a recent trend in the study of social movements, what Ingalsbee (1993) has referred to as a shift towards 'the semiotics of collective action', or what many others have referred to, simply, as the 'turn towards culture'. This turn towards culture is reflected in the work of leading scholars in the field and by the growing number of books and collections of essays that incorporate cultural factors and analyses into the study of social movements (cf. Ferree and Martin 1996; Johnston and Klandermans 1995; Laraña, Johnston and Gusfield 1994; McAdam, McCarthy, and Zald 1996; Morris and Mueller 1992). These volumes open new ground for theorizing and research, but they do so by moving in different directions.

Culture has most often been conceptualized within social movements theory in terms that emphasize its mental and cognitive dimensions. This tends to be true whether the object in question has been conceptualized using Marxist terminology as consciousness or ideology, as the collective identities of symbolic interactionists and 'new social movements' theorists, or as the discourses of cultural and postmodern theory. The concept that I use – cultures of action – expands the focus from the realm of disembodied cognition to include the emotional and physical dimensions of social movements. As such, my approach to studying culture is most indebted to the analytic insights and conceptualizations that have been developed in scholarship on practices and performance. Several contributors to *Social Movements and Culture* (Johnston and Klandermans 1995) analyse culture from this performative and practice-oriented angle.

In an essay entitled 'Cultural Power and Social Movements' Swidler (1995) synthesizes developments within cultural theory and social movements scholarship and affirms that social movements 'are the sites where new cultural resources, such as identities and ideologies, are most frequently formulated' (p. 30). She notes that 'altering cultural codings is one of the most powerful ways social movements actually bring about change' (p. 33), and that, because most movements lack political power, 'they can reshape the world more effectively through redefining its terms rather than rearranging its sanctions' (p. 34). Swidler argues that cultural theory is a rich source of insights for the study of social movements, but she also cautions against the tendency of social movements researchers to rely on a Weberian approach that locates culture in the thoughts, ideas and worldviews of individual activists. While acknowledging that this approach is easier for researchers to work with and operationalize, she points out that 'cultural theory is moving in the other direction' (1995: 31). Drawing on the work of Foucault (1977, 1980, 1983), Bourdieu (1977, 1984) and others, Swidler argues that an abundance of work now indicates 'that culture should be seen as socially organized practices rather than individual ideas or values, that culture can be located in public symbols and rituals rather than in ephemeral subjectivities, and that culture and power are fundamentally linked' (1995: 31). Swidler summarizes these developments in cultural theory as a shift towards thinking about culture in terms of 'publicness, practices, and power' (1995: 27).

This shift towards publicness, practices and power is evident in several other essays in this volume (Fantasia and Hirsch 1995; Fine 1995; Jenson 1995; Lofland 1995; Taylor and Whittier 1995). These contributors theorize social movements as staging areas for the production of culture, as contested terrains infused with power relations, and as sites in which discourses and symbolic objects are continuously negotiated, transformed and contested. Drawing upon Swidler's and others' insights, I have focused on public events and analysed these public events as ritualized performances. In doing so, I pay attention to the narrative conventions and discursive practices that feature prominently within them and I observe the ways in which these rituals function to produce and transform the emotions that create solidarity and strengthen participation (Fine 1995; Jenson 1995; Lofland 1995; Taylor and Whittier 1995). My study of the local terrain of breast cancer activism similarly embraces a tendency to shy away from removing culture from context, frames from feelings, and discourses from practices. However, I also seek to push this one step further. Re-embedding culture within context, frames within feelings, and discourses within practices allows the body – as a site of cultural contestation, a flexible signifier of identities and meanings, a vehicle for the expression of emotion, and an anchor of political logics – to emerge more clearly into the field of analytic vision. By incorporating the body into the study of culture and social movements, I seek to flesh out the disembodied conceptions of culture that define much of social movements scholarship. Thus, in the analysis that follows, I pay explicit attention to the ways that social movement culture is not only enacted, enunciated and emoted, but also, and importantly, embodied.

The San Francisco Race for the Cure®[4]

Background

The Susan G. Komen Breast Cancer Foundation, inventor of Race for the Cure, was established in 1982 by Dallas socialite Nancy Brinker and named in honour of her sister, Suzy, who died from breast cancer in 1980 at the age of 36. Two years after founding the organization, Nancy Brinker was herself diagnosed with breast cancer. But Brinker was luckier than her sister. She became a 'breast cancer survivor' and remained the driving force behind the Komen Foundation.

The Komen Foundation has played a paradoxical role in the breast cancer movement, acting as both a ground-breaking pioneer and a force of conservatism. In the early 1980s, at a time when no other nonprofit organizations were focusing exclusively on breast cancer, Nancy Brinker mobilized her tremendous economic, social and political capital to raise money for the promotion of breast cancer research and early detection campaigns. Brinker and the Komen Foundation thus carved out a new terrain for breast cancer advocacy and played a pioneering role in helping transform breast cancer from a hidden and unspeakable disease into a household word, a corporate language, a social problem and a legislatable issue. On the other hand, the Komen Foundation has adopted an uncritical stance towards the medical and research establishments – raising money for them, but never challenging their authority or priorities. And while the Komen Foundation has been at the forefront of redefining cultural meanings and representations of women with breast cancer, they have done so by tying these to norms of white, heterosexual, middle-class, consumerized femininity.[5]

Although the national organization has its headquarters in Texas, a network of volunteers working through local chapters spans the United States. The San Francisco chapter was formed in 1987. It was not until 1991, however, that the Komen Foundation became an important source of local funding. In 1991, San Francisco became one of 15 cities to host Race for the Cure. The San Francisco Race raised $232,000 and these funds were used to support biomedical research and to launch a programme, administered by the University of California, San Francisco, of mobile mammography vans that provide free screening to 'the medically underserved' (Chater 1992). Since 1991, the Race has been held annually in San Francisco, and biomedical research and early detection have remained the core mission of the local chapter, as well as the national organization. In October 1996, as part of National Breast Cancer Awareness Month, the sixth annual Race for the Cure was held in San Francisco's Golden Gate Park. The event drew almost 9,000 participants and raised over $400,000 (*San Francisco Chronicle*, 21 October 1996).

The 1996 Race for the Cure

It is a beautiful October morning in San Francisco. In Golden Gate Park, the atmosphere of a carnival prevails. The sixth annual Race for the Cure, sponsored by the Susan G. Komen Breast Cancer Foundation, is coming to life. Corporate booths line the outskirts of Sharon Meadow. Inside the booths, staffers display their wares. Dressed in running attire, thousands of women, children and men meander about. The crowd is about 75 per cent white and 75 per cent women, most of whom are toting clear plastic Vogue bags that contain free hair products, cosmetics, lotions and perfumes. The bags are rapidly filling up with more free items – pins of the newly issued breast cancer awareness stamp, pink ribbons and breast self-examination brochures. *Tropicana Orange Juice*, one of the national sponsors of the Race, offers some encouraging news about how to avoid breast cancer. We're told: 'Don't gamble with the odds. If you play it smart, you can beat them.' *Tropicana* even provides a sheet of diet tips and orange juice recipes to help us do it. The brochure explains that being overweight and not getting enough vitamin C are 'risk factors' for the development of breast cancer. Individual risk factors and breast health practices are consistent themes throughout the Race.

In addition to the booths of the corporate sponsors (*Chevron, Genentech, JC Penny, American Airlines, Ford, Pacific Bell, Vogue, Nordstrom, Wells Fargo, BankAmerica*), the medical care industry is in attendance, among those represented are: Kaiser Permanente, California Pacific, Davies Medical Center, UCSF-Mount Zion, the UCSF Mobile Mammography Van, and Marin General Hospital. In an increasingly competitive industry, women with insurance are a market that no one can afford to ignore. And in the breast cancer capital of the world, breast cancer is a big ticket item for the health-care industry.[6] The last few years have witnessed a whirlwind of sales, closures and mergers, and the medical centres that remain have reorganized their services and repackaged their messages better to appeal to the concerns and demands of female baby-boomer consumers. Old-fashioned hospitals and general medical centres have been replaced by women's health centres, breast health and breast cancer centres and the less specialized, more old-fashioned cancer centres. One breast health centre distributes an 11-page handout listing 34 services, groups and programmes for women with breast cancer and 'breast health' concerns.

Last but certainly not least, the fitness, nutrition, beauty and fashion industries are here in abundance. They offer an amazing array of services and top-of-the-line accessories tailored to the special needs of women in treatment for cancer and women who have survived breast cancer treatment. There are nutrition consultants, fitness experts and hair stylists. There are special lotions and creams. There are special swimsuits, wigs, scarves, make-up, clothing and vitamins. There are customized breast prostheses beginning at $2,100 and created from a cast of a woman's breast before it is surgically removed. There are partial prostheses for women with less radical surgeries. For the physically active crowd, there are sports bras, biker pants and baseball caps, with or without attached ponytails. There is sexy lingerie and lots of it. And in a stroke of marketing genius, a women's fashion catalogue weds the breast cancer patient's pursuit of femininity to the baby boomers' feminist sensibilities. The catalogue cover features a quote attributed to Simone de Beauvoir: 'One is not born a woman, one becomes one.' Inside are the means of (re)becoming a woman:

prostheses, lingerie, ponytails and fitness wear. This is the style of embodiment that is given centre stage at the Race.

Adding to the festive atmosphere are the shiny new automobiles parked in the middle of the meadow, adorned with balloons, courtesy of *Ford* and *Lincoln-Mercury* dealerships – national sponsors of the Race. In every direction, purple and aqua balloons dance in the air. Also bobbing about in the crowds and easily spotted from a distance, are women in bright pink visors. These visors signal a special status and are worn with pride. On each visor, below the corporate logos, the following message is stitched in black: 'I'm a survivor.' The visors are distributed from a special booth, situated in the centre of the meadow, the Breast Cancer Survivors' Station. Here, more than a dozen queues have formed with women standing six deep, chatting, socializing and awaiting their turn to receive the complimentary pink visor that marks them as a breast cancer survivor. As each woman dons her visor and mingles with the crowd, she proudly, voluntarily and publicly marks herself as a breast cancer survivor, visually embodying an identity not otherwise apparent. This is an act of social disobedience, a collective 'coming out', a rejection of stigma and invisibility, and a simultaneous appropriation of the traditional colour of femininity for the survivor identity. Later, after the Race has been run and walked, there is an official ceremony during which all the breast cancer survivors who wish to be recognized are asked to ascend the main stage. They are honoured for their courage in fighting breast cancer and for their willingness to demonstrate to other women, through their rejection of the cultural code of silence and invisibility, that breast cancer is not shameful, that it is survivable, and that it is neither disfiguring nor defeminizing.

One way of publicly remembering and honouring women with breast cancer is provided at the registration tables. Instead of the standard numbered forms pinned to the contestant's back, participants can choose to wear 'In Honour of' and 'In Memory of' forms displaying the names of women, both living and dead, whom they wish to honour publicly and acknowledge or mourn and remember. Like the visors, these forms are pink and they mark their wearers with a particular status. In choosing to display these forms, the participants identify themselves as part of the expanding circle of those whose lives have been touched by breast cancer. These moving displays generate powerful effects and enhance the intensity of the experience of moving en masse through the park with thousands of strangers to raise money for breast cancer. One encounters these pink signs here,

there and everywhere. The practice of wearing a sign is a way of enacting community, including oneself, in this sea of runners who have
suffered at the hands of this disease and who are working together to
raise awareness of breast cancer and money for mammograms and a
cure. They are powerful visual reminders of the pervasiveness of this
disease. These signs, like the visors, signify the public display of
private losses and triumphs. Wearing them is an emotional act at once
painful, brave and hopeful.

There are three more ways in which breast cancer is visually coded,
packaged and displayed. All three are stationed at one end of the
meadow, apart from the booths. The first display is in the form of a
large vertical cloth banner. The banner is imprinted with thousands of
pink ribbons – the symbol of breast cancer awareness. Many of these
ribbons are filled in with handwritten names. Everyone is invited to
write a name on a ribbon. The second display is 'The Breast Cancer
Quilt'. Modelled after the AIDS Quilt but in smaller dimensions, each
quilt – and there are several on display – contains approximately
twenty 12 × 14-inch panels. Unlike the AIDS quilt, which recognizes
those who have died, the Breast Cancer Quilt recognizes survival. Each
panel is created by a breast cancer survivor, or by a women who, at
least at the time of the quilt-making, was still a survivor. Not far from
the Breast Cancer Quilt is the 'Wall of Hope'. This display contains a
long series of panels. Each panel is comprised of fifteen 8 × 10-inch
'glamour photos' of breast cancer survivors. The survivors are
photographed in full make-up and adorned in brightly coloured
evening gowns, sparkling jewellery and even feather boas. Most of the
survivors are white. Women of colour stand out in a sea of light faces,
their visages poorly captured by a photographer accustomed to
working with lighter hues. Each woman is identified by name and
year of diagnosis or number of years of survival. Frozen in time, all of
these women are survivors, even those, unidentified, who are now
dead.

The message of the official programme, conducted on stage by a
woman in a pink visor, is clear and concise: the solution to breast
cancer lies in two directions, biomedical research and early detection.
The audience is informed that the Komen Foundation, sponsors of
this Race and 66 others being organized by local chapters throughout
the country, has contributed more money for breast cancer research,
screening and early detection than any other private organization
dedicated solely to breast cancer in the world. The audience learns
that the Susan G. Komen Breast Cancer Foundation was established in

1982 by Nancy Brinker in memory of her sister, Suzy, who died from breast cancer at age 36. 'Back then', says the speaker, 'there was no follow-up therapy, no radiation, no chemotherapy, no pill.'[7] Those were the dark ages of medicine.

The speaker continues with her story of individual control and medical progress: Nancy Brinker learned from her sister's experience 'that early detection is the key'. This knowledge served her well. As a result, she was vigilant and proactive in her own 'breast health practices' and was soon thereafter diagnosed with early-stage breast cancer. She is now a survivor. This is a story of success. The speaker concludes: 'This is what every woman here needs to know. All women should get a baseline mammogram at age 35, every two years after age 40, and yearly after age 50. And every woman should practise monthly breast self-exam.' The message here is clear: biomedical research has led to advances in breast cancer treatments that, in combination with breast self-examination and mammography are saving a new generation of breast cancer patients and transforming them into breast cancer survivors.

This is the archetypal story of Race for the Cure and National Breast Cancer Awareness Month. It is a story of individual triumph and responsibility. There is nothing sad or tragic about Brinker's encounter with breast cancer. Rather, her story is a narrative of unqualified success. It is also, of course, a story of failure and in this sense it serves as a cautionary tale. Suzy was not aware of, or did not practise, early detection. Suzy's breast cancer was diagnosed too late. She did not have access to radiation and chemotherapy. She died. In this morality tale the proactive survive and only the unaware and the irresponsible die. Responsibility exists solely within the context of detection, not within the context of causation. In fact, questions of causality are unspeakable in the terms of this discourse. In the discourse of the Race, survival is a matter of individual choice and responsibility. Regular mammograms never fail to diagnose breast cancer early and women diagnosed early never die.[8] For those who practise breast health, breast cancer may constitute a momentary setback but it is not a debilitating, recurring or chronic disease. In the discourse of the Race, breast cancer is part of each survivor's historical biography. A finished chapter. In this discourse, breast cancer is a disease of universal, individual, ahistorical, resilient, reconstructable, heterofeminine, biologically female bodies. Thus, the story told by Race for the Cure and enacted by the participants gathered together is a story of individual control and survivor pride, a narrative of hope, and a declaration of faith in the steady progress of science and medicine.

In addition to breast cancer survivors, there is a second category of women who are singled out for special attention. These women are constituted as 'the medically underserved'. Although the medically underserved are not visibly marked or present at the Race, except as signified indirectly by the UCSF Mobile Mammography Van, they are discursively constituted in official Komen publicity (brochures and registration forms) and by speakers who refer to programmes supported by money raised by the Race. Still, it is not clear who they are or why they are medically underserved. Like the simultaneously individualizing and universalizing category of the breast cancer survivor, the medically underserved are not situated as members of particular racial, ethnic, cultural, social, sexual, generational or geographic categories or communities. In the biomedical discourse of the Race, the medically underserved are represented as individual women whose needs can be met and managed by mammograms and breast health education.

The Bay Area Women & Cancer Walk

Background[9]

In the summer of 1991, three white lesbians, recent immigrants to the Bay Area, organized the first meeting of the Women & Cancer Project. The inspiration for this meeting, and the genesis of the cancer project itself, came from several places: the organizers' histories of involvement in feminist, and lesbian and gay communities; the recent cancer history of one of the organizers; and the powerful example and inspiration provided by the San Francisco gay community's ability to rally around and organize services for people with AIDS. The gay community's remarkable mobilization around AIDS led all three women to question the absence of a parallel mobilization around women's health. They saw that breast cancer was gaining ground in the media but, at the same time, nothing seemed to be happening in their community – no fundraising, no activism, no attention.

The first meeting of the Project included representatives from an array of women's health organizations whose foci ranged from breast cancer exclusively to women's health more generally. Representatives from Breast Cancer Action, the Women's Cancer Resource Center, the National Latina Health Organization, the Bay Area Black Women's Health Project and the Vietnamese Community Health Promotion

Project were present at the first meeting. Thus, from the beginning, an explicitly 'multicultural' vision and network informed the development of the Women and Cancer Project; and, although breast cancer was the starting point, from the beginning it was linked, both discursively and organizationally, to cancer as a broader category, and to women's health more generally.

The first Walk was held in 1992 and it has been held on an annual basis ever since. Every year proceeds from the Walk are divided evenly among the beneficiary organizations. Proceeds have ranged from a 1995 high of $7,000 per organization ($115,000 total raised), to a 1996 low of $2,500 for each organization. By 1995, the number of beneficiary groups had grown from six to 13. The steering committee, in theory comprised of at least one volunteer representative from each beneficiary organization, was in reality made up of whoever could come to meetings and work on the event. In practice, most of the volunteer labour and leadership was performed by a handful of white women who were connected to grassroots cancer organizations. The project has teetered on the edge of collapse for the last few years; despite having been established for some time, a consistent, reliable, template of systematization and procedure has not quite emerged. With no permanent paid staff or office space, rotating fiscal sponsors, low levels of institutionalization and organization, and the work burden carried by a few volunteers, most of whom are working full-time jobs elsewhere and are perpetually on the brink of burnout, every year the wheel, to some extent, must be reinvented.

Many of the walking teams hail from feminist or lesbian organizations and small, progressive businesses, and many of the individual supporters and volunteers also come from these networks and connections. But the project has been unsuccessful in more effectively harnessing the resources of these communities; and, although there is a great deal of discussion about tapping into the resources of the gay male community, with a few notable exceptions this has not happened. Yet another problem has to do with publicity and media messages. Many of the organizations do not focus specifically on cancer because they address the broader health needs of their communities. The Walk, in turn, has had difficulty developing effective ways of framing its focus and philosophy. Although in AIDS organizing it is common to fund community-based organizations that provide community-based, direct services and advocacy, the discursive terrain of breast cancer, its 'universe of political discourse' (Jenson 1987), has been effectively colonized by the discourses of research and early detection. The Walk has been unable effectively to communicate an alternative vision. Despite these obstacles, the actual number of participants in the Women & Cancer Walk has grown steadily, if slowly, each year, with many returning and familiar faces.

The 1996 Women & Cancer Walk

It is a crisp autumn morning in San Francisco. Gradually a crowd of between 600 and 800 assembles in front of a temporary stage in Golden Gate Park. This is the fifth annual Women & Cancer Walk. Like Race for the Cure, this is a fundraiser; but whereas the Komen Foundation funds biomedical research and screening mammograms for medically underserved individuals, proceeds from the Women & Cancer Walk support the work of a multicultural set of grassroots women's health and advocacy organizations. The Women & Cancer Walk takes place in the same meadow as Race for the Cure, and like the Race, it seeks to create a festive atmosphere; but the same meadow that held 9,000 participants and scores of booths and displays seems almost empty with fewer than 800 participants, a modest stage, a few folding tables and colourful splashes of artwork here and there. Neither balloons nor pink ribbons are in abundance. There is no sign of pink visors.

Like the Race, the Walk constructs and celebrates a particular symbolic community. But the symbolic community constructed by the Walk is quite different from that of the Race. The beauty, fashion and fitness industries are absent. So too, for the most part, is the healthcare industry. Instead, the community is comprised of dozens of volunteers, performers, speakers, walkers and the thirteen beneficiary organizations. The beneficiaries include three feminist cancer organizations and six women's health advocacy organizations: two Latina, two African American, one Vietnamese and one older women's. It also includes three community health clinics – one lesbian, one Native American and one serving a cross-section of poor people in San Francisco's Mission neighbourhood. But, although the Walk tries to construct a multicultural and multiracial community, the links within this community are visibly weak. Several of the beneficiary organizations are present in name only.

Like the Race, women, and white women in particular, predominate at the Walk. Many of the women here, however, hail from a different social location. Certainly, there are women here who would blend in easily at the Race, but they are neither the most visible nor the majority. At the Walk, there is a broad range of non-normative 'corporeal styles' (Butler 1990: 272) on display that, together, create a different kind of body politic. Though there are certainly active and athletic women in this crowd, they do not set the standard. Soft bodies in comfortable shoes replace hard bodies in exercise attire. There is a strong lesbian, feminist, queer and counter-cultural presence. It is signalled by styles of dress, hair and adornment; by the decentring of normative heterofemininity and the visibility of queer and lesbian relationships and sexualities. At the Walk, there are women with disabilities, large women, women for whom walking a mile will be an effort and for whom running a race would be out of the question. There are women with body piercings and tattoos. There are women with dreadlocks, short hair and no hair at all.

Hair provides an interesting twist on standards of deviance and normality. Whereas at the Race, companies market feminine wigs, scarves and hats to women seeking to disguise the effects of chemotherapy, at the Walk women who have lost their hair *involuntarily* blend in with women who have cropped their hair or shaved their heads *deliberately*, as part of a lesbian and/or queer aesthetic. The line between health and illness is more difficult to discern in a context where, instead of donning wigs to blend into the dominant norms of femininity, the norms are reconfigured so that bald women and women with very short hair move from the margins to the centre and women with carefully coifed corporate styles appear unusual.

On the other hand, there are women at the Walk whose breast cancer histories set them apart from other women in ways that are visible to the discerning eye. Whereas at Race for the Cure the identities of breast cancer survivors are stitched in black upon the bills of their pink visors, the breast cancer histories of some women at the Walk are inscribed upon their bodies in a way that is at one and the same time more subtle and, for many, more disquieting. Beneath their shirts it is possible to discern the outline of one breast, but not two. These women are not wearing breast prostheses and they have not undergone surgical reconstruction. Theirs is a doubly loaded act of defiance. Not only are they rejecting the code of invisibility, but the way in which they are doing so directly challenges dominant norms of beauty, sexuality and femininity. And it disrupts, quite visibly, attempts to tie the discourse of survival to the display of unmarred bodies.

This form of body politics is carried still further by RavenLight, an exhibitionist, sex radical, lesbian, feminist and cultural worker. RavenLight describes her work as 'educating the s/m community about breast cancer and educating women with breast cancer about sexuality'. At the Walk she is wearing a skin-tight black and white dress, black hose and high heels. Hardly the picture of normative femininity, however, one half of her dress is pulled downward and secured at the back, starkly revealing the evidence of her breast cancer history. The smooth, pale surface is exaggerated by the fullness of her remaining breast. As I accompanied RavenLight on the one mile walk through the park, a woman in her late fifties approached us from behind. As she pulled up beside us and peered across, she exclaimed, 'Oh good! That's what I thought! Well then: I'm going to take my shirt off too!' She then removed the two shirts she wore that were covering a sleeveless, skin-tight, grey unitard that showed off the asymmetry of her chest and made it clear that she, too, had had a mastectomy. Here, in the context of the Walk and in the company of a fellow traveller, this woman was moved to reveal publicly her breast cancer history, to display an otherwise hidden form of embodiment and to celebrate an alternative style of femininity.

For the past couple of years, 'Walkers of Courage' have been named and honoured on stage. Sometimes they are women with breast cancer histories. Just as often they are women currently living with metastatic disease. But always, they are women who are singled out for their service and activism rather than for their survival. Last year Gracia Buffleben, a woman then living with advanced metastatic breast cancer, was honoured as a Walker of Courage. During the previous year, Buffleben and other breast cancer activists, following in the footsteps of Elenore Pred, one of the founders of Breast Cancer Action, had worked with AIDS activists to graft ACT UP tactics onto breast cancer activism. In December they had organized civil disobedience against Genentech, a powerful Bay Area biotech company, in order to win 'compassionate use' access to a promising new drug then in clinical trials. When Buffleben ascended the Women & Cancer Walk stage to accept her award, ACT UP activists, dressed in black, stood behind her holding signs with rows of gravestones. The signs read: 'Don't Go Quietly to the Grave. Scream for Compassionate Use!' In form and structure, this ceremony was no different from Race for the Cure's on-stage recognition of breast cancer survivors. The contrast in images and meanings, however, was telling: pink versus black; survival versus death; gratitude versus anger.

As in previous years, this year's programme is deliberately multicultural and multiracial – more so than the audience. Sign language interpretation is provided on stage. The pre-walk warm-up is led by an

Afro-Brazilian dancer and masseuse. The disc jockey is well known in the lesbian club scene. And live music is performed by an African-American woman and a white man who are local jazz musicians. The discursive performances are similarly diverse.

The first speaker, a Walk organizer, begins by noting that women's health concerns have been 'systematically ignored and underfunded' and that 'healthcare and social services are least accessible to the women who need them most.' At the same time, the speaker notes, cancer rates have continued to rise to epidemic proportions and 'one in three women will be diagnosed with cancer in her lifetime'. This is the same discourse that circulates on the pledge sheets and event programmes. It broadens the terms of the discourse from breast cancer to all cancers that affect women, and from breast cancer early detection to broader concerns about women's health and access to health care.

Next, San Francisco Mayor Willie Brown gives a brief speech. This is the first time that a politician of such stature has addressed the Women & Cancer Walk and it is not entirely clear how the audience feels about his presence. The Mayor affirms his commitment to solving the problem of breast cancer and he publicizes and promotes the forthcoming Mayor's Summit on Breast Cancer. Then, misjudging at least part of his audience, he slides seamlessly into a soundbite on prostate cancer and reminds the audience that men get cancer too, and that he intends to address the growing problem of prostate cancer. Some women in the audience applaud. Others hiss and shake their heads. The woman I am standing next to, a member of staff at a feminist cancer agency, turns to me, rolls her eyes and says: 'Does he have any clue about the issues? Does he have any idea who he's talking to? Does he realize that this is the *Women* and Cancer Walk!?'

One of the two main speakers is the director of the Native American Health Center in Oakland. She begins by speaking about the devastation of the environment and its negative impact on the well-being of the earth and all of its inhabitants. She speaks about the large Native American community in Oakland that she belongs to and describes the lack of access to basic healthcare services and cancer support programmes. She then describes the uses to which the money donated to her health centre by the Women & Cancer Walk has been put. These funds paid for the cab fare to the hospital for a woman receiving chemotherapy but too sick to take the bus across town. It paid for the phone service for a woman dying of cancer so that she could talk to her family in the southwest during her final weeks. It bought Christmas toys for the children of a third woman with cancer. It paid for therapy for a fourth woman, also dying; and it helped pay her funeral expenses. Each woman's story is narrated with compassion and respect.

These are stories of desperation, hardship, loss and death. The subjects of these stories do not speak for themselves: they are spoken of, but they are spoken of, and discursively constituted, as women with complicated commitments and biographies, as women with their own needs, histories, priorities and desires. They are individuals, but individuals embedded within particular cultures, communities and institutionalized inequalities. These women are not passive, but certainly they are victims – victims of multiple institutionalized inequalities – and cancer is just one of many obstacles that they are up against. Perhaps some will become long-term survivors, but this is not where the logic of the narrative leads. This is a narrative of harsh realities, poverty and dislocation, not a discourse of individual choice and responsibility, or hope and triumph.

Although the Women & Cancer Walk focuses on services and advocacy for women with cancer, in recent years it has joined this to an environmental justice discourse of cancer prevention. This year the final speaker is an Italian woman who has never been diagnosed with cancer but who is an environmental activist and crusader for cancer prevention. She delivers an impassioned speech that at key moments elicits enthusiastic applause from the audience. She weaves together the global connections between rising cancer rates, profit-driven industries and environmental racism.

The Toxic Tour of the Cancer Industry

Background[10]

In the summer of 1994, a handful of Bay Area activists convened an informal meeting to network, learn about each other's work, identify areas of overlap and explore the possibility of working together on issues of mutual interest. These activists came from four organizations: Breast Cancer Action, Greenpeace, West County Toxics Coalition and the Women's Cancer Resource Center. At their second meeting, they decided to formalize the collaboration and named themselves the Toxic Links Coalition (TLC). The formation of the Toxic Links Coalition thus represented a local synthesis of the feminist cancer and environmental justice movements, which has grown to include more than 20 organizations.

During the first two meetings, as they shared information and educated one another, they decided to focus their energies on challenging the pristine image and hegemonic discourse produced and circulated by National Breast Cancer Awareness Month (NBCAM). Invented in 1985 by the London-based Imperial Chemicals Industry (ICI) and later taken over by its subsidiary, Zeneca Pharmaceuticals, NBCAM was viewed by these activists as a wolf in sheep's clothing: a public relations campaign that expanded the market for treatment drugs and detection technologies, legitimized early detection programmes as the only conceivable public health approach to breast cancer, and effectively concealed from the public the fact that multinational corporations, assisted by their allies, were profiting by *causing* cancer on the one hand, and detecting and treating it on the other. In other words, as TLC activists would say, 'they getcha coming and going'.

The basis of these claims was simple. Zeneca Pharmaceuticals not only funds and controls the publicity for NBCAM's breast cancer early detection campaigns, but they also, through their parent company ICI, manufacture pesticides and herbicides that contribute to causing it. Adding more fuel to the fire, Zeneca is the manufacturer of tamoxifen (brandname Nolvadex), the world's best-selling breast cancer treatment drug (categorized by the World Health Organization as a carcinogen) and the owner of Salick, Inc., a management company that runs a dozen cancer treatment centres across the country – including a cancer centre just down the road from the TLC meeting place. ICI/Zeneca/NBCAM/Salick thus represented a textbook case of vertical integration. And every October, through a series of public and private partnerships and in combination with hundreds of thousands of posters, pamphlets, radio spots, newspaper ads and promotional videos, NBCAM promoted the message that 'Early detection is your best protection.' Neither the word 'carcinogen' nor 'cause' had ever appeared in NBCAM publicity.

NBCAM thus seemed the perfect target. Its discourse of early detection and its refusal to speak of carcinogens and prevention was understood by TLC activists as a campaign of miseducation, obfuscation and shameless profiteering. Therefore, as part of their project of re-education, the TLC declared that October was no longer National Breast Cancer Awareness Month but was instead renamed Cancer Industry Awareness Month. TLC's first collective action was to set up an informational picket at the 1994 Race for the Cure in Golden Gate Park. They targeted the Race because its sponsor, the Komen Foundation, was a participant in NBCAM and because the Komen

Foundation, like NBCAM, avoided any mention of causality, carcinogens or the environment in its publicity. This action was followed, within a couple weeks, by the first Toxic Tour of the Cancer Industry; invented by the TLC, the Cancer Industry Tour quickly became the signature of this group and the focus of their energy in years to come.

The 1996 Cancer Industry Tour

It is noon on Wednesday, and in downtown San Francisco a crowd has gathered on Market Street, in front of Chevron's corporate headquarters. Metal barriers and uniformed police line the sidewalk and street for about 100 feet, separating the courtyard, sidewalk and street traffic from the protesters who are assembling inside the barriers. A large banner identifies the coordinators of the event. It reads 'Toxic Links Coalition – United for Health and Environmental Justice'. Another large banner reads 'Stop Cancer Where It Starts!'. The demonstrators begin walking in an elongated circle, carrying signs aloft and loudly chanting 'Stop Cancer Where it Starts! Stop Corporate Pollution!' 'Toxins Outside! Cancer Inside! Industry Profits! People Suffer!' and 'People Before Profits!'.

The 1996 Cancer Industry Tour is the third annual event and it draws approximately 150–200 participants. As in previous years, the Toxic Tour is designed as a one-hour *tour de force* that moves through downtown San Francisco and stops at specific 'targets' along the way. The 1996 targets are *Chevron*, *Pacific Gas & Electric*, Senator Dianne Feinstein, Burson Marsteller (a public relations firm), *Bechtel* (builder of nuclear power plants) and the American Cancer Society. The Cancer Industry Tour shifts the focus even further away from the universal, feminine, individual frames of Race for the Cure. Although the Tour is similar to the Walk in that many of the speakers locate themselves as members of particular communities, in the Toxic Tour, the focus of their political discourse shifts *away* from their community and group identities in order to constitute and draw attention to the local outposts of the global cancer industry.

The theme of the Tour is 'Make the Link!' and the Tour is choreographed so that each stop along the way represents a link in the chain of the cancer industry. TLC publicity materials assert that 'the cancer industry consists of the polluting industries, public relations firms, [and] government agencies that fail to protect our health, and everyone that makes cancer possible by blaming the victims and not addressing the real sources.' This is a smear campaign, a strategy of public shaming, an attack on corporate images. At each stop a culprit is identified and their name is bellowed out over a bullhorn. A description of corporate practices destructive to human health and the environment follows. Literally and figuratively, the cancer industry is mapped through the delivery of speeches, the display of props and signs, and the movement from site to site. The speakers call for a politics of cancer prevention and an end to environmental racism.

There are clear lines separating 'them' from 'us', and those lines are reinforced by the uniformed police escort and barricade. This is street theatre. It is ritualized confrontation and condemnation. And it creates opportunities for the mobilization and expression of oppositional identities. Like the Race and the Walk, about three-quarters of the participants are white and three-quarters are women, but many – perhaps a half – of the authorized speakers are people of colour, both women and men. They speak not as individuals, but as members and representatives of environmental justice organizations. There are also speakers from feminist cancer organizations – Breast Cancer Action, the Women's Cancer Resource Center, Impart, Inc. (a breast implant activist organization) and individual activists living with cancer. All of the speakers express anger, outrage and injustice, and these emotions are mirrored and affirmed by the Toxic Tour participants. Although some speakers identify themselves as 'living with cancer' and 'breast cancer survivors', many do not. Like the Race and the Walk, men are in the minority at the Tour. But unlike the Race and the Walk, men speak from positions of entitlement equal to those of the women speakers. There are no men, however, who identify themselves as cancer survivors or living with cancer and speak from either of those subject positions.

This is not primarily an expression of solidarity with, or sympathy for, people with cancer. It is a collective expression of rage at the cancer industry's destruction of the health of all people, but particularly those living in communities affected by environmental racism. Like the Race and the Walk, breast cancer occupies a privileged position in speakers' narratives and in the visual signs and signifiers. But just as the Walk decentred breast cancer by connecting it to other forms of cancer that affect women, the Toxic Tour decentres breast cancer by linking it to cancers affecting men, women and children, and further still, to a host of environmentally related health conditions such as reproductive, respiratory and autoimmune diseases. In this context, everyone is part of the inner circle of the aggrieved; but it is not grief that is mobilized, it is anger.

The bright orange flyers distributed along the way announce that one-third of American women and one-half of American men will be diagnosed with cancer in their lifetime. It states that the lifetime risk for breast cancer is 1 in 8 and rising, that the Bay Area has the highest rates of breast cancer in the world; and that African-American women living in Bayview-Hunters Point, a low-income and predominantly African-American community, have breast cancer rates double that of the rest of San Francisco (see Jennifer Fishman's chapter in this volume). The orange flyer also states that 'we are all exposed in increasing doses to industrial chemicals and radioactive waste *known* to cause cancer, reproductive, and developmental disorders' and that 'big profits are made from the continued production of cancer-causing chemicals'.

Last year, the 60 or so protesters carried handmade signs painted with slogans, miniature coffins and gravestones emblazoned with a handwritten name, a lifespan and the letters 'RIP'. This year, there are more than twice as many participants as last year and the coffins and gravestones are nowhere to be seen. Instead, two show-stealing props have appeared: The first prop is a gigantic puppet with moving arms, deftly operated by a team of three. The 20-foot puppet is a papier-mâché woman with blue skin and a mastectomy scar dripping blood where her second breast should be. In each of her gigantic moveable hands she holds a container of toxic substances, painted with a skull and crossbones. The second prop is a tall, narrow float on wheels, one side of which is painted as a man in a business suit, but without a head; the other side of the float is a skyscraper with an assortment of corporate insignias: *Chevron, PG&E, Dow, Dow Corning, Monsanto, UNOCAL, US Ecology*. This float is known as the Tower of Evil. Images of death, deformity and destruction abound at the Toxic Tour.

One woman holds high an exhibit of photographs of women's nude torsos. They include startling images of disfigured women with double mastectomies – some of them with the concave chests characteristic of the Halsted radical mastectomy, a particularly mutilating and in some cases debilitating surgical procedure performed by American surgeons from the 1880s until the 1980s. Other women distribute vivid colour photographs of ruptured implants and mutilated chests – the result of negligence on the part of Dow Corning, Inc., the manufactures of silicone implants. It is just these sorts of images that Race for the Cure seeks to banish from the collective consciousness. But here they are resurrected and pasted onto sandwich boards and donned by angry women marching through downtown San Francisco.

There are no freebies distributed at this event: none of the beauty products, pink ribbons or breast health brochures that abound at the Race. There are no corporate sponsors. Although Chevron and the American Cancer Society are present at both the Race and the Tour, they are participants and sponsors of the Race whereas they are targets of the Tour. At the American Cancer Society, for example, Judy Brady, a breast cancer activist and self-described 'cancer victim', delivers a series of withering accusations which she substantiates by distributing copies of a recent internal ACS memo marked 'Confidential'. The memo comes from the national office and instructs local offices to ignore and suppress a brochure on cancer and pesticides created and distributed by a small office in the Great Lakes region. She charges the ACS with miseducating the public, ignoring cancer prevention, refusing to take a stand against industrial and agricultural pollution, and colluding with the corporate stakeholders to hide evidence of corporate carcinogens. Brady's assertion of her identity as a cancer victim is laden with significance. It reclaims a highly stigmatized identity that the breast cancer survivor identity was designed to displace. At the same time, it resignifies this identity by disconnecting it from earlier associations with passivity and connecting it instead to a confrontational politics. The association with victimization is deliberately reasserted, but instead of being victimized by a random, terrorizing disease, the person with cancer is resituated as a victim of the brutal cancer industry.

At the Toxic Tour, there is no call for more research to uncover the mysteries of tumour biology or discern the patterns of cancer epidemiology. There are no visions of more or better science, or for more or better social and medical services. There is no call for women to be vigilant, to practise breast self-examination and get mammograms. Mammography *is* invoked, but as an example of false promises and corporate profiteering. These activists do not promote the ideology of early detection. They do not promote the notion that disease growing within community bodies can be mapped onto the genetic structures and 'risk factors' of individual lifestyles. 'Cancer', they stress, 'is not a lifestyle choice.' Instead of mapping the biomedical geography of individual women's bodies and behaviours, as in the Race, or mapping the social geography of communities and health services, as in the Walk, the Toxic Tour maps the political economy and geography of the cancer industry – the hidden maze of linkages and networks connecting the bodies of state agencies, politicians, charities and profit-driven corporations to the unhealthy bodies of people involuntarily exposed to toxins and living in contaminated communities. The

Toxic Tour maps the sickness and disease of toxic bodies and the body politic onto the corporate corpus. Cancer prevention, they make clear, requires a different kind of cartography.

Comparative Summary and Theoretical Implications

Each of these three social movement events was designed to educate and motivate, to 'raise awareness' and mobilize action. The concept of 'cultures of action' (Lofland 1995) is used here to develop a comparative, descriptive analysis of differences within the field of breast cancer activism in the San Francisco Bay Area. First, whereas Race for the Cure singled out breast cancer, the Women & Cancer Walk expanded the category to include all cancers affecting women, and the Toxic Tour of the Cancer Industry expanded the category still further, to include cancer in general and other environmentally related diseases. Second, whereas the Race drew upon biomedicine and represented breast cancer as a universal, ahistorical disease of biologically female bodies that could be controlled through salvationist science, surveillance medicine and individual vigilance, the Walk drew upon multicultural feminism and represented cancer as a body-altering, life-threatening source of suffering that was compounded by institutionalized inequalities in access to healthcare and social services. The Toxic Tour, on the other hand, drew upon the environmental justice movement and discourses of environmental racism to represent breast cancer as the product and source of profit of a predatory cancer industry. In Race for the Cure, the most privileged and honoured identity was that of the breast cancer survivor. The Women & Cancer Walk, on the other hand, created more space for the identities of women 'living with cancer' and women dying from the disease. Finally, the Toxic Tour decentred women as a category, gender as a lens of analysis and even, to some extent, the identities of participants altogether. Instead, the Toxic Tour highlighted the identities and relationships of specific industries and organizations, and discursively constituted, from these linked identities, an entity that they named the cancer industry. Finally, the Race called for more biomedical research and early detection, and supported the provision of mammograms to the medically underserved; the Walk called for better healthcare and social services, and supported the work of community clinics and women's health advocacy and activism; and the Toxic Tour called for cancer prevention instead of early detection, for more corporate regulation instead of more research, and supported the work of coalition members on behalf of environmental health and justice.

All three social movement events produced and promoted different cultures of action not only by enunciating them, but by physically enacting them. Clearly, the activities of *racing* for the cure for breast cancer, *walking* for women with cancer and *touring* the cancer industry are symbolically laden, but part of this symbolic charge came not just through naming and framing, but through physical participation. Participation in collective action, after all, is a physical and emotional experience as well as a cognitive and mental one – and the latter may well be balanced on the knees of the former. Consciousness, ideologies, mentalities, discourses and collective action frames are enabled not simply through abstract mental processes, but through practices of participation that work on and through bodies. Indeed, as Louis Althusser wrote, quoting Pascal, 'Kneel down, move your lips in prayer, and you will believe' (1970: 168).

In terms of emotional expression, also an embodied experience, all three events mobilized feelings of togetherness and solidarity. But beyond this, they diverged. The Race mobilized hope and faith in biomedicine, while also mobilizing the respect of Race participants *for* women with histories of breast cancer and mobilizing self-pride *among* breast cancer survivors. The Walk, on the other hand, mobilized anger against the same institutions celebrated and trusted by the Race, the institutions of biomedicine and the healthcare system. At the same time, the Walk mobilized respect for the work of cancer activists and women's health organizations, and privileged the identities of women dealing with cancer – but it did so by positioning them as fighting and suffering women, rather than as victors who believed they had defeated breast cancer and put it behind them. Finally, the Toxic Tour mobilized a deep sense of injustice and choreographed the expression of anger and outrage against the cancer industry and its destruction of human health and the environment.

Each culture of action represented breast cancer through the lens of a particular conception of the body, and in each case this corporeal model was reinforced by particular corporeal styles. The Race, ironically enough, embraced a corporeal model that the cancer historian Robert Proctor (1995) has referred to elsewhere as 'body machismo'. Proctor uses this term to illustrate the tendency of industry allies and anti-environmentalists to conceptualize the human body as a 'macho body' that is able to withstand repeated environmental insults, detoxify potential carcinogens and repair genetic damage (1995: 171). Race for the Cure, interestingly enough, promoted a feminized and domesticated version of this 'macho body' and connected it to medical technologies rather than environmental carcinogens. In Race for the Cure the macho body morphed into the heterofeminine, resilient body: the repaired, reconstructed body beautiful, responsive to medical treatment and safe from the spectre of recurrence. The corporeal styles that were produced and promoted at the Race were those that represented and reinforced this corporeal model: unmarred bodies, fitness activities, visually marked survivor identities and the reassertion of heteronormative femininities. Thus, in the context of the Race, the absent breast was flawlessly concealed by prostheses and reconstructive surgeries and the only indication that breast cancer could result in altered bodies was found in the corporate booths, where wigs and prostheses circulated as free-floating commodities.

The corporeal model undergirding the analysis of the Toxic Tour of the Cancer Industry, on the other hand, embraced what Proctor has termed 'body victimology' (1995: 171). This corporeal model focuses on the vulnerability of the body to toxic assaults and its weakness in the face of repeated exposures to carcinogens. Indeed, some cancer activists in the Toxic Tour directly challenged the implicit corporeal model of the breast cancer survivor identity and explicitly asserted the identity of cancer victim. In turn, the victimized body was visually represented at the Tour through pictures of mutilated bodies, ruptured implants, props with mastectomy scars dripping blood, canisters of poison, RIP signs and coffins. At the Toxic Tour, the vulnerable, victimized body was represented in the form of death and mutilation.

The Women & Cancer Walk also embraced a corporeal model of body victimology, but it developed a different variation on this theme. In the case of the Walk, it was the physical effects of cancer treatments that were represented through the visual display of altered bodies. In the Walk, cancer recurrences and metastases were not banished from the collective consciousness, and health and recovery were represented as tentative and possibly temporary. Here, women living with cancer could feel comfortable not concealing their chemically and surgically altered bodies. Here, the absent breast was actually 'present' as an absence, directly challenging the corporeal model of resilient, reconstructed bodies and the display of unmarred bodies. The subtly altered bodies of the Walk also posed a challenge to the Toxic Tour's representation of the victimized, graphically mutilated body. And even RavenLight's overtly exhibitionist style of body activism drew attention to the sexuality and beauty of one-breasted women and mobilized pride and self-acceptance. She did not represent herself as victimized and mutilated, and the mastectomy scar she exposed was thin and healed, not the gory and mutilating scars on display at the Toxic Tour. Thus, as in the case of the Race and the Toxic Tour, the Walk's political vision was anchored in a set of interpretations of women's bodies and these interpretations were mobilized and reified through different styles of embodiment.

Until recently, the hegemonic model for interpreting and acting with regard to breast cancer, in the United States, has been the biomedical model developed by scientific medicine and delivered by the healthcare industry. Race for the Cure, while embracing many of the assumptions and visions of this biomedical perspective, was able to challenge successfully some of its stigmatizing practices and effects by redeeming and revalorizing the social identities of women with breast cancer. The biomedical model has been challenged in more radical ways, however, by the local women's cancer movement and by the environmental justice movement. The women's cancer movement, represented by the Women & Cancer Walk, challenged the narrowness of the biomedical model by insisting that the problems of breast cancer be examined from a wide-angle lens that extended beyond the parameters of the clinic and screening procedures and into the communities in which women actually live, and struggle to live, with cancer post-diagnosis. The Toxic Tour of the Cancer Industry, the synthesis of the feminist cancer community and the environmental justice movement, challenged the biomedical model from a different angle. Whereas the Walk directed attention beyond the medical clinic and drew attention to struggles and problems that occur *after* the moment of diagnosis, the Toxic Tour redirected the focus to a point in time *before* the moment of diagnosis and *before* the practices of screening and early detection. The environmental justice movement, represented by the Toxic Tour, reframed the agenda around the politics of cancer *prevention*. In so doing, however, the needs of women actually living with breast cancer were pushed back into the margins.

The cultures of action created and deployed in the Women's Walk and the Toxic Tour of the cancer industry have been misrepresented and ignored by dominant media representations of the breast cancer movement. They have been silenced and dismissed by the state, the healthcare system and the forces of corporate capital. By amplifying the voices and making visible the cultures of action that have been minimized by dominant representations, I have sought here to recover some of these 'subjugated knowledges' (Foucault 1980) and to represent some of the 'stories less told' (Darnovsky 1992). At the same time, I am also interested in drawing attention to aspects of culture within social movements that have received short shrift within the sociological literature. Here, too, there are subjugated knowledges and stories less told, and these stories have to do with the ways that meanings are not only collectively enacted and enunciated, but are shaped and informed by profoundly emotional and embodied dimensions of experience and participation. Thus I have attempted here to complicate narratives of the breast cancer movement and, at the same time, to complicate sociological narratives of culture within social movements. This is accomplished by paying attention to the ways in which bodies figure not only as sites of disease, but as the vehicles and products of social movements, and as anchors and signifiers of contested meanings.

Acknowledgement

I thank the individuals and organizations, both named and unnamed, who participated in the events and movements written about here. Their visions and commitment inspired my analysis and I hope they will see themselves reflected in this text. I also thank Michael Burawoy and the Global Ethnographies Group for their valuable comments and criticisms on a different version of this essay, and for helping me figure out, with both patience and exasperation, what it is I'm trying to say, even as it changes: Joseph A. Blum, Teresa Gowan, Sheba M. George, Lynne Haney, Séan O'Ríain, Millie Thayer, Zsuzsa Gille and Steven Lopez. Thanks also to Barrie Thorne, Raka Ray, Arlene Kaplan Daniels and the editors and anonymous reviewers of *Social Problems* for their thoughtful comments and suggestions. Finally, I thank the Berkeley Department of Sociology and the Barbara Rosenblum Scholarship for the Study of Women and Cancer for their generous support of this research. Earlier versions of this paper were presented at the World Conference on Breast Cancer in Kingston, Canada (July 1997) and at the Annual Meetings of the American Sociological Association in Toronto, Canada (August 1997).

An extended version of this chapter was published in *Social Problems*, vol. 46, No.1, and we thank The University of California Press for permission to reproduce the work here.

Notes

1 Some of the factors that distinguish recent forms of cancer activism from those of the past are: 1) the fragmentation of the category of cancer into the narrower and more specialized categories of particular *types* of cancer; 2) the movement of *breast* cancer, in particular, into a politically and discursively privileged position; 3) the prominence of new subjectivities and collective identities (e.g., breast cancer survivors, breast cancer warriors, women living with cancer; women at risk); and, 4) the scale and scope of activism and the density of networks and linkages between proliferating organizations, campaigns and coalitions.

2 More than three years of participant observation in the San Francisco Bay Area began in the autumn of 1994. Field research included the observation of four different cancer support groups (ranging from two months to two years), ongoing volunteer work at a feminist cancer resource centre, and participant observation in a range of networks, projects, fundraisers, cultural events, educational forums, environmental protests, street theatre, public hearings, early detection campaigns, and various conferences and symposia. My research also included more than 40 taped interviews with cancer and breast cancer experts, advocates and activists. Although this paper grew out of a broader framework of fieldwork, it draws most directly upon my participant observation of the three events in question – Race for the Cure®, the Women & Cancer Walk and the Toxic Tour of the Cancer Industry. I conducted participant observation at four consecutive Race of the Cure events held in San Francisco (1994–7), I helped organize and staff two Women & Cancer Walks (1995–6), and, I also participated in three consecutive Toxic Tours of the Cancer Industry (1995–7) and attended TLC meetings beginning shortly after the group's formation in 1994.

3 This identification of commonalties is accomplished in different ways, and with different purposes, in each of the three studies under discussion. Montini (1996) creates a category comprised of a representative sample of women activists from each of the states that attempted to pass breast cancer informed consent legislation. She then uses grounded theory to analyse her interview data and looks for what is common, or generalizable. Taylor and Van Willigen (1996) use diverse sources of data to develop an analysis of the breast cancer movement as a whole so that they can position it and the postpartum depression movement as representative of self-help movements in general. They, like Montini (1996), look for commonalties and generalizable characteristics rather than dissimilarities and distinctions. Anglin (1997) positions her case study of a breast cancer organization as representative of the breast cancer movement as a whole. She then develops a critique of the movement by drawing upon texts produced and circulated within arenas outside of it.

4 'Race for the Cure' is a registered trademark. For the sake of easier reading, I have eliminated the trademark symbol (®) in the remainder of the text.

5 For example, Brinker and the Komen Foundation pulled out of the committee that issued the call for, and guided the formation of, the feminist National Breast Cancer Coalition. One interview subject told me that, at this meeting, 'the Komen ladies, dripping in diamonds, sat on one side

of the table, and across from them were some women from the Mary Helen Mautner Project for Lesbians and Cancer.' According to the story told by this interviewee – a story I have often heard repeated in activist circles – the Komen ladies (and they are always referred to as 'ladies') decided to pull out of the NBCC as it was in the process of formation because they did not want to work with feminists and lesbians. The repetition of this narrative within certain networks speaks to a particular set of cultural and political divisions that the Komen Foundation is seen as representing.

6 For the past 20 years, the San Francisco Bay Area has had the highest documented rates of breast cancer in the world. The figures available in 1994 showed that the rate was 'about 50% higher than in most European countries and five times higher than in Japan' (Northern California Cancer Center, 1994).

7 'The pill' refers to tamoxifen, a hormonal, systemic treatment for women who have been diagnosed with breast cancer (and approved in September 1998, by the FDA as a 'preventative' treatment for healthy women at 'higher risk' for developing breast cancer). Although the speaker at the Race referred to the early 1980s as a time when neither tamoxifen, chemotherapy nor radiation were available to women with breast cancer, this is not entirely accurate. All three treatment modalities were available and used during the early 1980s, although tamoxifen and chemotherapy were typically reserved for women with later stage disease (De Gregorio and Wiebe 1994; Moss 1995). But the details and accuracy of the speaker's narrative are less important than the trope of medical progress.

8 According to even the most conservative estimates, mammograms (and the radiologists who interpret them) fail to diagnose breast cancers large enough to be visualized by this technology at least 15 per cent of the time – even more among premenopausal women ('Fact Sheet on Breast Cancer', Office of Women's Health, U.S. Public Health Service, n.d.). Most breast cancers do not appear on mammograms and cannot be 'seen' by radiologists until they have been growing for about eight years (Love and Lindsey 1995: 265).

9 The historical data for this background section are based on an interview (1997) with Abby Zimberg, one of the founders and key organizers of the Women & Cancer Walk. The rest of the analysis is based on my participant observation of organizing meetings and activities during 1995 and 1996, and my participant observation during the actual events.

10 The information about the first two meetings of the Toxic Links Coalition (TLC) is based on interviews with the cancer activist Judy Brady and the public recounting of this history at various events. I began doing participant-observation of the TLC in the early stages of its formation in October 1994, so most of this information comes from my notes on those meetings and from early events, including the 1994 demonstration at Race for the Cure.

References

Agran, L. *The Cancer Connection – And What We Can Do About It* (Boston, MA: Houghton Mifflin 1977).

Althusser, L. *Lenin and Philosophy and Other Essays* (New York: Monthly Review Press 1971).

Altman, R. *Waking Up, Fighting Back: The Politics of Breast Cancer* (New York: Little, Brown and Company 1996).

Anglin, M.K. 'Working from the Inside out: Implications of Breast Cancer Activism for Biomedical Policies and Practices'. *Social Science and Medicine* 44 (1997) 1403–15.

Batt, S. *Patient No More: The Politics of Breast Cancer* (Charlottetown, Canada: Gynergy Books 1994).

Bourdieu, P. *Outline of a Theory of Practice* (Cambridge: Cambridge University Press 1977).

Bourdieu, P. *Distinction: A Social Critique of the Judgment of Taste* (Cambridge, MA: Harvard University Press 1984).

Brady, J. ed. *1 in 3: Women with Cancer Confront an Epidemic* (San Francisco, CA: Cleis Press 1991).

Breslow, L. and D.M. Breslow. 'Historical Perspectives on Cancer Control'. *Readings in American Health Care: Current Issues in Socio-Historical Perspective,* ed. W.G. Rothstein (Madison, WI: University of Wisconsin Press 1995) pp. 364–74.

Butler, J. 'Performative Acts and Gender Constitution: An Essay in Phenomenology and Feminist Theory'. *Performing Feminisms: Feminist Critical Theory and Theatre*, ed. S.E. Case (Baltimore, MA: The Johns Hopkins University Press 1990) pp. 270–82.

Carson, R. *Silent Spring* (New York: Houghton Mifflin Company 1962).

Chater, V. 'The Run of Their Lives'. *Northern California Woman* (October 1997).

Clorfene-Casten, L. *Breast Cancer: Poisons, Profits and Prevention* (Monroe, ME: Common Courage Press 1996).

Colborn, T., D. Dumanoski, and J.P. Myers. *Our Stolen Future: Are We Threatening Our Fertility, Intelligence, and Survival? – A Scientific Detective Story* (New York: A Dutton Book 1996).

Darnovsky, M. 'Stories Less Told: Histories of US Environmentalism'. *Socialist Review* 22 (1992) pp. 11–54.

Enrique, L., H. Johnston and J. Gusfield, eds. *New Social Movements: From Ideology to Identity* (Philadelphia: Temple University Press 1994).

Epstein, S. *The Politics of Cancer* (Garden City, NY: Anchor Books 1978).

Fantasia, R. and E.L. Hirsch. 'Culture in Rebellion: The Appropriation and Transformation of the Veil in the Algerian revolution'. *Culture and Social Movements*, eds. H. Johnston and B. Klandermans (Minneapolis, ME: University of Minnesota Press 1995) pp. 144–62.

Ferraro, S. '"You Can't Look away Anymore": The Anguished Politics of Breast Cancer'. *New York Times Magazine* (15 August 1993) pp. 24–7, 58–62.

Ferree, M.M. and P.Y. Martin, eds. *Feminist Organizations: Harvest of the New Women's Movement* (Philadelphia: Temple University Press 1995).

Fine, G.A. 'Public Narration and Group Culture: Discerning Discourse in Social Movements'. *Culture and Social Movements*, eds. H. Johnston and B.

Klandermans (Minneapolis: University of Minnesota Press, 1995) pp. 127–43.

Fosket, J., C. LaFia and A. Karran. 'Breast Cancer in Popular Women's Magazines from 1913 to 1996'. *Breast Cancer: The Social Construction of Illness*, eds. S.J. Ferguson and A.S. Kasper (New York: St. Martin's Press forthcoming).

Foucault, M. *The Birth of the Clinic: An Archaeology of Medical Perception* (New York: Vintage Books 1973).

Foucault, M. *Discipline and Punish: The Birth of the Prison* (New York: Vintage Books 1977).

Foucault, M. *History of Sexuality*, vol. 1 (New York: Pantheon Books 1978).

Foucault, M. 'Two Lectures'. *Power and Knowledge: Selected Interviews and Other Writings 1972–1977*, ed. Colin Gordon (New York: Pantheon 1980) pp. 78–108.

Foucault, M. 'Afterword: The Subject and Power'. *Michel Foucault: Beyond Structuralism and Hermeneutics*, eds. Hubert Dreyfus and Paul Rabinow (Chicago: University of Chicago Press 1983) pp. 208–26.

Ingalsbee, T. 'Resource and Action Mobilization Theories: The New Social Psychological Research Agenda'. *Berkeley Journal of Sociology* 38 (1993) pp. 139–56.

Jenson, J. 'Changing Discourse, Changing Agendas: Political Rights and Reproductive Policies in France'. *The Women's Movements of the United States and Western Europe: Consciousness, Political Opportunity, and Public Policy*, eds. M.F. Katzenstein and C.M. Mueller (Philadelphia: Temple University Press 1987) pp. 64–88.

Jenson, J. 'What's in a Name? Nationalist Movements and Public Discourse'. *Social Movements and Culture*, eds. H. Johnston and B. Klandermans (Minneapolis: University of Minnesota 1987) pp. 107–26.

Johnston, H. and B. Klandermans, eds. *Social Movements and Culture*, vol. 4 (Minneapolis: University of Minnesota Press 1995).

Kushner, R. *Breast Cancer: A Personal History and an Investigative Report* (New York: Harcourt Brace Jovanovich 1975).

Kushner, R. *Alternatives* (Cambridge, MA: The Kensington Press 1984).

Linden, R. 'Writing the Breast: Contests over Screening Mammography, 1973–1995'. *History and Philosophy of Science Colloquium*. Stanford University (27 April 1995)

Lofland, J. 'Charting Degrees of Movement Culture: Tasks of the Cultural Cartographer'. *Culture and Social Movements*, eds. H. Johnston and B. Klandermans (Minneapolis: University of Minnesota Press 1995) pp. 188–216.

Lorber, J. *Paradoxes of Gender* (New Haven, CT: Yale University Press 1994).

Lorde, A. *The Cancer Journals* (San Francisco, CA: Aunt Lute Books 1980).

Love, S. with K. Lindsey. *Dr. Susan Love's Breast Book*, 2nd edn (New York: Adison-Wesley Publishing Company 1995).

Markle, G.E., J.C. Petersen and M.O. Wagenfeld. 'Notes from the Cancer Underground: Participation in the Laetrile Movement'. *Social Science and Medicine* 12 (1978) pp. 31–7.

McAdam, D., J.D. McCarthy and M.N. Zald. 'Opportunities, Mobilizing Structures, and Framing Processes: Toward a Synthetic, Comparative Perspective on Social Movements'. *Comparative Perspectives on Social*

Movements: Political Opportunities, Mobilizing Structures, and Cultural Framings, eds. D. McAdam, J.D. McCarthy and M.N. Zald (New York: Cambridge University Press 1996).

Melucci, A. 'Paradoxes of Post-industrial Democracy, Everyday Life and Social Movements'. *Berkeley Journal of Sociology* 38 (1994) pp. 185–92.

Montini, T. 'Women's Activism for Breast Cancer Informed Consent Laws'. Unpublished doctoral dissertation. University of California, San Francisco, 1991.

Montini, T. 'Gender and Emotion in the Advocacy of Breast Cancer Informed Consent Legislation'. *Gender and Society* 10 (1996) pp. 9–23.

Morris, A. and C.M. Mueller, eds. *Frontiers in Social Movement Theory* (New Haven, CT: Yale University Press 1992).

Moss, R.W. *The Cancer Syndrome* (New York: Grove Press, Inc. 1982).

Moss, R.W. *Questioning Chemotherapy* (New York: Equinox Press 1995).

Northern California Cancer Center. 'Greater Bay Area Cancer Registry Report' 5(1) (1994).

Office on Women's Health. 'Fact Sheet: Breast Cancer'. U.S. Public Health Service: Washington D.C., distributed at Women's Health and Emerging Issues: California Perspective conference; co-sponsored by California Public Health Association-North and the Office of Women's Health, California Department of Health Services (24 October 1997)

Patterson, J.T. *The Dread Disease: Cancer and Modern American Culture* (Cambridge, MA: Harvard University Press, 1987).

Paulsen, M. 'The Politics of Cancer'. *UTNE Reader* (November/December 1993).

Paulsen, M. 'The Cancer Business'. *Mother Jones* (May/June 1994).

Proctor, R.N. *Cancer Wars: How Politics Shapes What We Know and Don't Know About Cancer* (New York: Basic Books 1995).

Rennie, S. 'Mammography: X-rated Film'. *Chrysalis* 5 (1977) pp. 21–33.

Rettig, R.A. *Cancer Crusade: The Story of the National Cancer Act of 1971* (Princeton, NJ: Princeton University Press 1977).

Ross, W.S. *Crusade: The Official History of the American Cancer Society* (New York: Arbor House 1987).

San Francisco Chronicle. Bay Area Section (21 October 1996): C1.

Soffa, V.M. *The Journey beyond Breast Cancer: Taking an Active Role in Prevention, Diagnosis, and Your Own Healing* (Rochester, VT: Healing Arts Press 1996).

Stacey, J. *Teratologies: A Cultural Study of Cancer* (New York: Routledge, 1997).

Steingraber, S. *Living Downstream: An Ecologist Looks at Cancer and the Environment* (New York: Addison-Wesley Publishing Company 1997).

Stocker, M. ed. *Cancer as a Women's Issue: Scratching the Surface*, vol. 1 (Chicago: Third Side Press 1991).

Stocker, M. ed. *Confronting Cancer, Constructing Change: New Perspectives on Women and Cancer*, vol. 2 (Chicago: Third Side Press 1993).

Swidler, A. 'Cultural Power and Social Movements.' *Social Movements and Culture*, eds. H. Johnston and B. Klandermans (Minneapolis: University of Minnesota Press 1995) pp. 25–40.

Swidler, A. 'Culture in Action: Symbols and Strategies'. *American Sociological Review* 51 (1995) pp. 273–86.

Taylor, V. and M. Van Willigen. 'Women's Self-help and the Reconstruction of Gender: The Postpartum Support and Breast Cancer Movements'.

Mobilization: An International Journal 1 (1996) pp. 123–43.

Taylor, V. and N. Whittier. 'Analytical Approaches to Social Movement Culture: The Culture of the Women's Movement'. *Social Movements and Culture*, eds. Hank Johnston and Bert Klandermans (Minneapolis: University of Minnesota Press, 1995) pp. 163–87.

Yadlon, S. 'Skinny Women and Good Mothers: The Rhetoric of Risk, Control, and Culpability in the Production of Knowledge about Breast Cancer'. *Feminist Studies* 23 (1997) pp. 645–77.

4
Publishing the Personal: Autobiographical Narratives of Breast Cancer and the Self

Laura K. Potts

Over the last ten years or so, a number of personal accounts of the experience of having breast cancer have been published, many by women who would not previously have identified themselves as writers. I am interested here to consider the role and purpose of these narratives, and, in particular, to identify the ways in which they form some kind of metanarrative with common themes to the stories they tell, and the clear stylistic and political antecedent they evoke, in the form of consciousness-raising within the women's liberation movement. The texts raise a number of questions which will be addressed here: What role does storytelling have in contemporary Western culture for the writers and for the readers? To whom do the texts speak and what are their intentions? In what ways are the narratives told, and how do these processes inform our understanding of autobiography as a genre? Finally, the articulations of the self, and the use of narrative to make sense and meaning of experience will also be examined, in the context of contemporary feminist philosophies of subjectivity.

The 1990s may be characterized by a dominant culture of revelation, disclosure and the making of testimony through a variety of media, and the more recent of these texts may be shaped by that currency of trend. As a set of texts, however, they are also informed by the long tradition of autobiographical writing and its 'valorization' of a life, as Stanley (1992) has it. A diary style is the most favoured form for these stories, characteristically both intimate and private; within the genre of disease stories, even more than in other types of women's autobiographical writing, there is 'public acceptance of the right of the autobiographer to satisfy her own needs in writing' (Lury 1987: 58). It is held to be a good and healthy thing to do: good for the writer, a process of catharsis, and good for the reader too, to learn and to empathize; this is 'the political and therapeutic power of personal story-telling' of which Jo Spence speaks (Spence 1995: 133). The diary style sets few constraints on the writer, sanctioning stylistically free self-expression, and establishing, by its immediacy and implication of authenticity, an authority which makes the texts hard to question. The narratives are not readily contestable, and indeed the orthodoxy of such testimonials demands the reader's belief and acceptance of what she is told. (This too was a feature of consciouness-raising, and one which mired feminist debate in epistemological confusion: women's accounts were presented as uncontestable knowledge. 'That's how it felt so that's how it was.') In this way, then, the texts are authoritative and claim to present truths about the author; they are intended to be directly referential of her life, as well as literary constructs. In some cases this makes for uncomfortable reading; the detail of Jenny Cole's (1995) daily living with her cancer and the confusion she experiences yields a text that is charged with all the muddle, anxiety and obsessiveness that she describes. Reading it, I longed for a little distance, to be able to stand away from her life and her story. No doubt she felt the same.

Both with and for Others

A privileged access to intimate and very personal stories of another's life was an integral tenet of the Women's Health Movement in the 1970s and 1980s, as part of a conscious and radical determination to name and expose the socially constructed and punishable shameful-ness of all aspects of female embodiment (thanks to Maren Klawiter for this reflection). In open defiance of the postmodern thesis and its assertion of the redundancy of the author *qua* person, Kearney (BBC Radio Three, 4 October 1996) stated that one of the tasks of narrative remains that of offering exemplars; the participation of the reader in the narrative provides the possibility of a sense of shared humanity. Similarly, Stanley claims of autobiographical narratives in particular that readers read 'these because in a myriad of ways' they have 'rever-berations for how we understand our own lives, experiences, times' (1992: 99). The poet Joolz said (in performance, Spring 1997) that we tell stories to bind us together, so that neither the listeners nor the tellers feel alone. While Joolz's comment related to the face-to-face and oral storytelling which is her work, certainly it usefully describes too the feminist project of consciousness-raising in the second wave (and arguably since time immemorial in a less formalized sense), and which is illustrated by these texts too.

By telling our experiences we hear them in new ways: by listening to the tales of others we are able to make connections with other women's lives and so to make a new sense of what we feel and what we are living through. The revolutionary potential of consciousnness-raising (c.r.) was the granting of political significance to personal experiences, the way in which insights gained from the discussion and illumination of determining structures gave a different and shared meaning to what had seemed to be isolated and discrete, so that a new sense of self might emerge, connected to those other sisters with whom the process was shared. It seems to me that similar processes are revealed by the texts studied here. Several of them describe the author's search for other women who had had breast cancer who could help them in their own understanding. Batt (1994: 22) says, 'I want to know their stories', and that she read Rose Kushner (1975)- one of the earliest personal testimonies of breast cancer – like 'listening to a big sister who's been there'; Mayer (1993: 73) also tells of how she wanted stories, other women's memoirs of their 'inner lives', to help her make sense of her own experience/story. She does this in response to her feeling of alienation from the normal world and writes of the 'information and comfort' she finds in talking to other women (*ibid.*: 47). The point is not to standardize the recounting or the experiencing of the lifestory, but to learn from the insights of others, to widen one's perspective and apply different ways of understanding. The same challenge is made to the reader of these narratives, whether she has breast cancer or not: How am I to respond to these stories? What is the point of reading of the harrowing traumas that another woman has lived through? Answering these questions leads at least in part to a reiteration of the political purpose of c.r.: we are bound to an understanding of another's experience, a connection that invites solidarity. There is little distance constructed between the writer and the reader; as Cole states, 'you know me' (Cole 1995: 382). And that knowing is an intense and intimate relationship, established through the exposure of 'private' traumas of body and mind, and by the immediacy of the favoured present tense. The uses of this close relation between writer and reader are integral to the political purposes which frame the narratives: having stepped into another's shoes, it is often not easy to kick them off again.

Audre Lorde writes her *Cancer Journals* to be 'of use', and 'for other women of all ages, colours and sexual identities who recognise that imposed silence in any area of our lives is a tool for separation and powerlessness' (1980: 9) and wants 'the record ... to be ... something that I can pass on' (*ibid*.: 46). Other writers similarly offer their stories as gifts to their readers: Cole (1995: 384) asks herself: 'do you want it published because of the glory attached to being a published author ... or do you want to offer help to others?', and answers herself: *'(To help others).'* Butler and Rosenblum write to provide 'a map' for other women – part of their intention is to be there as guides for other women: 'enter the world we inhabited together, to see parts of your-selves in us, and perhaps to live more fully and deeply because of all we learned' (1994: Introduction). Having looked for guides, these writers look to be guides: 'from woman and toward woman', as Cixous says (1989: 111). Her notion of the gift and of exchange in writing is useful in considering these texts: she is concerned to iden-tify the difference between the 'masculine profit' of man's writing and the 'economy of femininity' of woman's writing. 'All the difference lies in the how and why of the gift, in the values that the gesture of giving affirms, causes to circulate' (*ibid*.: 107). Here is how Lorde expresses that intention in her own work: 'May these words serve as encouragement for other women to speak and to act of our experi-ences with cancer and with other threats of death, for silence has never brought us anything of worth. Most of all, may these words underline the possibilities of self-healing and the richness of living for all women' (Lorde 1980: 10). The direct connection to the reader, and particularly to those readers who also have breast cancer, proposed by these texts manifests precisely the relationship that Cixous describes, of an 'open, extravagant subjectivity' (1989: 111). This is illustrated too by Mayer's closing pages (1993: 172-3), in which she describes how a friend sent her a stone from a beach, and imagines how 'later that day, she wraps up the stone to send it to me. She hesitates, and wonders if perhaps she should keep it for herself. Then she decides to send it after all.'

Collective Experience, both 'Shared and Unique'

The texts have a relationship to each other, then: they combine to form a coalition of insight and perspective that is stronger than the sum of its parts. Such a modification of the traditional masculine lifestory genre, with its emphasis on the accounting of/for an indi-vidual and frequently idealized life story, objectively constructed, yields a double stranding in these narratives. There is both the discrete and individualized experience of breast cancer, and the sense of it as a common and shared story. The sense of a collective narrative is not necessarily a joint project, but may rather be interpreted as a connective experience, both 'shared and unique' (Friedman 1988: 40). As Rosenblum says: 'without the historical frame of reference, my individual case suffers from lack of fuller meaning' (1991: 243); Butler and Rosenblum (1991: Introduction) claim that 'this is already a shared epidemic, a collective experience'. This poses a challenge to the dialectic of illness characteristic of dominant Western culture. On the one hand '[m]odern Western culture portrays people as private and bounded; consequently illness is seen principally as a problem of the individual' (Yardley 1997: 7). On the other hand, the discourses of epidemiology and of allopathic medical treatment tend to group all sufferers together into a homogeneous category defined by the disease. As Mayer comments (1993: 25), 'Medicine depends on our physical similarities, from which it draws its conclusions. The old truism from the anatomy lab still obtains: We are all the same under the skin.' Certainly, the experience of breast cancer is still 'lived through … other categories of identity and community', as Cartwright states and, as she asserts, 'to underscore the unifying factor of disease' is not unproblematic (1998: 119). In recognizing connectivity through these narratives, the individual is not effaced, but nor is the collective import of the shared story denied; that dialectic is resolved, the polarity of positions dissolved. But this is not to homogenize. This was the political significance of consciousness raising, too.

The narratives thus confirm the accuracy of some feminist critiques of auto/biographical theory, as it has traditionally related to male lifestories: Friedman, for instance, sees Gusdorf's classic analysis of autobiography as stressing 'individualistic paradigms' and ignoring 'the role of collective and relational identities in the individuation process of women' (1988: 35). 'Isolate individualism is an illusion,' she asserts (*ibid.*: 39), and certainly her thesis would seem to be supported by the very connectiveness and interdependency that these texts reveal. The narratives, then, do not position themselves as representative, but rather assert what Waugh (1996: 341) defines as the 'collective relational subjective', a recognition that each of us is not uniquely and originally situated. This is despite what Flax calls the 'specifics of location and participation' (Flax 1990: 293). Her notion of a project to retell and reconstruct women's 'differentiated but collective experience' (*ibid.*) is realized in these texts in a demonstrably political manner too, as Susan Love's afterword to Walder's story emphasizes. 'Joyce Walder has written "My Breast" as "One Woman's Story", but it is a story that has become far too common. It is a story of many women, young and old, poor and well-to-do, black and white. It is a story of an unmarried forty-four-year-old career woman in New York and of a married woman of thirty-five with young kids, living in the Midwest. It is the story of an elderly widow and a young lesbian' (Walder 1992: 167).

Certainly for the reader there is a commonality in the narratives, in the stories and the subject positions presented: women's experience of breast cancer is both personal and private, and collective and connective. As Lorde states, 'There is a commonality of isolation and painful reassessment which is shared by all women with breast cancer, whether this commonality is recognised or not' (Lorde 1980: 10). I think it is useful here to refer to Stanley's comments on 'the way in which a "self" is construed and explored as something more than "individual": unique in one sense, but also closely articulating with the lives of others' (1992: 14). This is no essentialized nor universalized merging of experience; it is generated initially by the association with other women, face to face or through their words, dissolving the 'isolation with my predicament' of which Mayer writes (1993: 74), and asserting 'this involuntary sisterhood' (*ibid.*: 4), as c.r. did. The location of personal experience in a social and political context is particularly evident in the work of Batt (1994), Spence (1995), Lynch (1986) and Lorde (1980), but it is the multigenred nature of Batt's text which most emphatically reveals a connection to other women with the disease, and an opening of the wider social context in which it is experienced. Recounting her story alongside the research she undertook, with the stories of other women's experiences to which that led her, yields a text which both asserts her self and positions her as part of a collectivity of women who have breast cancer in common. In this way the text provides what women may be fortunate enough to find in self-help groups. Lorde also establishes those connections, without denying the diversity of experience: 'Breast cancer and mastectomy are not unique experiences, but ones shared by thousands of American women. Each of these women has a particular voice to be raised in what must become a female outcry against all preventable cancers, as well as against the secret fears that allow those cancers to flourish' (Lorde 1980: 10).

Asserting the 'I'

Against this connectiveness, however, is set the isolation which all the writers describe. Here, for instance, is Lorde: 'Where are the models for what I'm supposed to be in this situation? But there were none. This is it, Audre. You're on your own' (Lorde 1980: 29). Writing in the face of this terrifying loneliness reveals what may seem at first paradoxical in the context of the preceding argument: facing the threat to the continuing reality of the self and the body that breast cancer poses, these women write to confirm their *individual* identities and their sense of self. And this practice sits comfortably within a classical masculine paradigm of autobiographical practice, defined as having 'a single, radical and radial energy originating in the subject center, an aggressive, creative expression of the self, a defence of individual integrity in the face of an otherwise multiple, confusing, swarming, and inimical universe' (Olney, quoted by Friedman 1998: 36). Significantly, the description of the universe used by Olney here resonates loudly with the dominant tropes of cancer mythology – of disorder, mystery, a body turned against itself, of uncontrollable replication of rogue cells. So while the texts tell a *shared* story, breaking down the isolation of the women's experiences of breast cancer with an assertion of the connective and collective, they also assert the unique and *individualized* self. Each of these narratives concerns a process of ordering the construction of self/new self through 'successive images, or still lives' as Gertrude Stein has it (Brodski and Schenk 1988:7) to 'fix and contain' not just the new identity she can find to be shared with others with breast cancer, but an individualized identity in the best liberal humanist tradition.

So I want now to examine this further feature of these texts, the way in which they assert the individual self, not in contradiction of what has previously been asserted regarding shared identity, but as the tying in of another strand to the whole. This too seems to reflect the process of feminist consciousness raising: how, in common with these narratives, it served to assert both a refashioning of the self through collective repositioning and the generation of new meaning; how the strength of a sense of sisterhood, or collective identity could, ideally, reflect a strengthened personal identity.[1] These autobiographical texts provide a legitimising location for what Judith Butler (1990: 143) calls an 'assertion of "I" ... the invocation of that pronoun', in a very materially substantive way. It is, after all, crucially an *individual* woman who faces this threat to her life. 'A load of survival is pulling you from your "you" of the dead, pushing it up to float outside you like an astral body. You try to get up. You are going to try in the First Person. Do "I" want to? "I" will try' (Julien 996: 75). The texts themselves, then, provide the structure of signification. This affirmation of the 'I' is crucial to the political purpose of these texts, women with breast cancer positioning themselves as they understand themselves, in public. As Brodski and Schenk state, 'the case of autobiography raises the essential problem in contempoary feminist theory and praxis: the imperative situating of the female subject in spite of the postmodern campaign against the sovereign self' (1988: 14). Even as the writers search for a location for themselves as women with breast cancer alongside other women with the disease and acknowledge the strength in that shared identity, they also recount the process of coming to a new personal identity too. The 'sovereign self' is as crucial to a feminist project as the 'collective' self; individual women's survival is important.

In Spence's poem *New Knots*, similar tensions are expressed as 'Questions of autobiography and authorship ... reworking those accounts ... The problem of being de-centred (that is having lost the idea of a coherent and autonomous self); how we are constructed across and between discourses (what about the bits in between?) ... the problem of being out of control in the present (destruction and rebellion in various discourses) ... illness: the ultimate crisis of self-representation' (Spence 1995: 146). Shildrick considers this 'whole set of troublesome issues concerning the deconstruction of subjectivity', and concludes, 'If the notion of a self-present, self-authorising subject, the "I" who speaks and acts, is put in doubt, then the issue of moral agency loses its transparency of meaning and the very focus of feminist enquiry dissolves' (Shildrick 1997: 128). In this context it is importantly not just moral agency that becomes meaningless, but the struggle to survive breast cancer as a disease and as a social process; in the face of a life-threatening disease, these narratives pragmatically emphasize the 'I' as present and actively engaged in living and challenging the loss of authority to the medical profession and to the disease itself.

So these narratives relate literally rather than only metaphorically to Cixous's project of the subversive feminine text: 'Write yourself: your body must make itself heard' (1989: 116). '[W]oman, writing herself, will go back to this body that has been worse than confiscated, a body replaced with a disturbing stranger, sick or dead, who so often is a bad influence, the cause and place of inhibitions' (*ibid.*). The act of writing is a crucial affirmation of living, a statement against fear-fulness, invisibility and silence, in Lorde's words (1980: 61). Yorke has written of this in relation to Adrienne Rich's poetry and essays of the 1970s; how she asserts the importance of speaking against erasure and silencing, speaking out from the silences that smother underlying terrors (Yorke 1998). Facing the threat of the ultimate erasure, 'the problem of final and total silence' (Spence 1995: 146), writing becomes a form of survival. 'Write or be written off', Spence titles a photo of herself hidden under/draped by a sheet on a narrow hospital like bed (*ibid.*: 100). 'My own writing has been a source of joy and nourishment to me', says Rosenblum in a letter to her friends (Butler and Rosenblum 1994: 166), and Butler says in her introduction that 'we wanted to tell our story, finally, because this writing made us visible to ourselves as we were living it' (*ibid.:* Introduction). Visible to the self through writing; visible to the world through publication: this is the 'transformation of silence into language', of which Lorde writes, the 'act of self-revelation' (1980: 21).

Making Sense, Making Meaning

Autobiography, as Duncker asserts, 'is often a search for coherence and explanation' (1992: 56). The telling of these stories takes on a further significance as the making of sense from the writer's experi-ence; as Lynch says in reply to a psychologist who asks her why she is writing about 'what it is like to have cancer', 'because writing is what I do. It helps me sort out ideas and emotions and find out what I really feel' (Lynch and Richards 1986: 35). This genre of narrative as self-discovery is familiar, a journey as Spence (1995) describes it, one in which the narrator/protagonist writes 'to sort out for myself who I was and was becoming at that time' (Lorde 1980: 53). Cole finds the 'meaning of my sickness through writing' (p. 201), a meaning she also hopes to discern from her exhaustive visits to a range of 'alternative' practitioners – the majority of whom offer explanation alongside treatment. Brohn (1987) takes a not dissimilar path, looking to make new sense of her life, to find meaning in the intervention of the disease as a significant and reappraised part of her experience.

The meaning of the disease is not, however, given with the diagno-sis of symptoms. Through the recounting of individual stories, the narratives serve to reinforce the multiplicity of meanings that breast cancer has, reminding us too that breast cancer is not just one disease, as campaign and promotional literature would have us believe. One

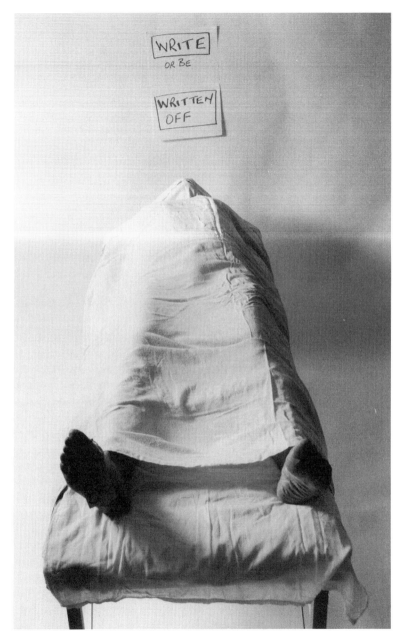

Figure 2 'Write or Be Written Off', 1998, by Jo Spence in collaboration with David Roberts (*Jo Spence Memorial Archive, London*).

function of self-help groups for women with breast cancer is the sharing of stories, an oral and interrupted version of the storytelling considered here. The telling of stories may also often concern the articulation of each participant's sense of the meaning of the disease to her, including what she has been told and what she has read, but also generating a sense of meaningfulness through the dialogic process. The meanings each woman ascribes to her breast cancer vary according to her social positioning, the other identities she has and the 'differentials of class, cultural identity, ethnicity and sexuality' (Cartwright 1998: 119). The crafting of the narrative becomes the crafting and ascribing of meaning to the experience of the disease and its effects on the life and the self.

In the narrativization of a life generally, and in the case of these texts in particular, what is additionally revealed by the process of literary construction is the meaning of a life – the meaning given to it by the narrator, at any rate. In writing or telling lifestories, 'it is the act of remembering, an act which is both critical, affirmative and selective, that places boundaries and edges around the story, giving it its seeming internal coherence' (Ahmed 1997: 162), This becomes the meaning of the narrative. But of course, as Culler points out, in reading a narrative 'readers and critics [do not] restrict themselves' to particular interpretations, nor even the preferred interpretation of the writer – there are 'competing theories of the meaning of works' from which we build our understanding (Culler 1981: 48). He questions whether the meaning in a narrative is shown to be an effect or a cause of the prior reported event (*ibid.*: 171); in the case of the texts studied here, the discursive presentation is actually predicated on the making of meaning, on making sense for themselves, quite clearly as an effect of the story. The act of writing is precisely concerned with the generating of meaning in the narrative; so Butler and Rosenblum state that their 'reflections were an attempt to fix meaning' (1994: Introduction), and Acker states that she writes to give meaning against the meaninglessness of the disease experience (1997).

The texts are thus constructed against one of the dominant experiential senses of the breast cancer, which are of disorder, the mysteriousness of causality (Batt 1996), the initial loss of previous meaningfulness and of uncontrolled growth (Sontag 1979). The meanings of a life, or of a disease, are not, however, either conclusive or all pervasive. The gaps and discomforts in Cole's account, for instance, provide an example of the 'contrary logic' to which Culler refers (1981: 175), denying the reader the pleasures of a coherent and unified account. Her narrative itself seems to reflect the uncertainty and confusion which characterize the 'story' of a cancer, and the way in which it is represented as something out of control, rampant within (Stacey 1997). Others write explicitly against this characterization: Julien (1996: 95) suggests that 'Perhaps I believed for a while – that ... my jabbering in the margin would capture what I couldn't work out (and what was frightening me) in this vertigo of an agony set in the present tense'. While the story of the woman may offer some attempted coherence and ordering, the disease story itself may be less biddable. So Spence writes of her leukaemia: 'This time around, I'm spending my time trying to decide what sort of story my illness is telling ME, rather than trying to impose a narrative onto other people that I still don't even understand myself' (Spence 1995: 216).

In generating meaning, the texts all provide some kind of protest against the normative construction of what a woman with breast cancer is like. Brohn (1987), for example, writes with a fervour to tell how having breast cancer can be approached to challenge the medical orthodoxy. And Mayer writes of the 'reframing of illness' in her text, against the dominant neat TV and magazine formulation of the 'problem of the week' (1993: 104) and 'beyond the usual inspirational memoirs ... and self-help nostrums for overcoming this or that difficulty in life' (*ibid.*: 6). This process can be understood, in Spence's words as: 'deciding to become the subject of our own histories rather than the object of somebody else's' (1995: 129). This radical, transformative potential has been identified by Edward Said (1978) in relation to colonial dominance and resistance, but it is equally applicable to the texts considered here, where the emphasis on the personal, individual and subjective (usually female) telling of a story of breast cancer is set against the authoritative, medical, expert voice (usually male). These women with breast cancer move through the boundaries and barriers of the medical profession and cancer industry, asserting their status as someone with authority in relation to their bodies and the disease (McRobbie 1994). Inevitably, this is not a comfortable process:

> I am furious. Disgusted. And I am really tired, tired of closed doors. Eighteen months of closed doors. Administrators, doctors, social workers – as concerned with hiding their own shortcomings as with easing cancer patients' burden. I am so sick of medical secrecies masking as rules and regulations. It seems I have come full circle. The writer who believed she had a heartwarming and urgent story to tell is still running into dead ends. (Lynch and Richards 1986: 141)

It is these dead ends which prompt the writing in many cases; the need to make sense, not just privately but in public, of the experience of the disease. And Lynch's weary irritation with the establishment is also voiced by other writers; the writing of their own account and own meanings becomes an important assertion of autonomy when the disease itself removes so much control.

In this context, then, what is important is that the women are all, in some way, writing against the 'dominant literary and political institutions which legitimate and reproduce the "master narratives" (Waugh 1996: 363), and against the 'prevailing social order' (Friedman 1998: 38). Of course, this has always been an important project for writing feminism, and in the work of the women's health movement too, which has consistently challenged the authority and the legitimacy of medical and professional voices and made opportunities for different narratives and different voices to be heard. These texts are variously positioned in relation to a literary or publishing world, and their authors' access to alternative forums in which to be heard vary a great deal too. Several already had a published authorial voice prior to their breast cancer and this particular narrativization: Spence was a photographer and activist/writer published in cultural journals; Lorde an acclaimed feminist writer and academic; Mayer had written a novel after completing a Masters programme in writing; Lynch, Batt and Walder all worked as journalists; Butler and Rosenblum were academics, and Segrave was an aspiring writer with friends in journalism. All cases of 'in and against the system'; as Waugh (1996) has argued, the position of women within these dominant institutions implies an inevitable tension. But there is undoubtedly an ease in their proximity to the means of publication, of getting their voice heard, even if this is not necessarily apparent in the text itself. The absence of that status is perhaps more marked: Cole's narrative recounts a struggle to be published alongside the other struggles with her disease and destructive personal relationships, and in this respect her book is exceptional – she has no previous history which might grant her a means of publication. It becomes a story that cannot be told by the dominant literary institution, one which has to be made public through different means.

The ways in which the texts are written against the norms vary widely. Stacey (1997) has shown how the dominant cancer narrative is one of heroism, of confronting the monsters, battling against the odds, and of triumph – a construction evident in a number of different genres, populist, medical and feminist. There is a trajectory in which the heroine emerges richer for her experience, a 'better person', the kind of woman we are all supposed to be, who copes with whatever life throws at her. In contrast, Spence describes her work, her writing and her photographic work, as 'unofficial storytelling' (Spence 1995: 135); it directly opposes the given reality, creating an alternative which is not shaped by the same old patterning, and yields for her the conclusion 'that I have not "arrived" anywhere' (*ibid*.). Many of these narratives reveal a variety of positions in relation to the normative construction of the cancer patient. Mayer, for instance, writes of 'putting up the brave front that was quickly becoming second nature', (Mayer 1993: 65), and characterizes herself as returning to a 'self I'd been struggling for years to overthrow ... the good little girl – no, more than good. Heroic' (*ibid*.: 76). But she also writes, within very few pages of these comments, of feeling 'neither brave nor optimistic, ... anxious ... out of control ... knocked off balance', and of how she 'was not inspired' by the models of women she has read about who have emerged 'victorious' over their cancer, or 'whose courage had stood fast through lingering, valiant deaths' (*ibid*.: 78). Like any norm, this has been internalized by its reinforcement in much of the literature of personal cancer testimony; it would be strange not to see it manifest at all in these narratives, whatever the intention to construct a different story. Cole (1995: 84) explicitly states that she wants to write in a way that does not speak of the bravery and courage in fighting the disease, and the voice she uses reveals a tortured and unresolved confusion that is not an acceptable or usual literary mode. (No doubt this explains the reluctance of any publisher to take her book on; her struggle and determination to be heard meant she had to publish the book herself.) But, none the less, she permits into the text other people's perceptions of her as a courageous fighter, and includes citations from her readers that testify to her power to inspire. To some extent, at least, it is attractive to be regarded as a heroic protagonist of one's own lifestory.

Ways of Telling: Narrative Form and Function

In terms of the dramatic potential of the telling of these stories, the texts frequently begin with a known ending – or at least the blurb on the back may tell us that the woman is still alive or dead. So we may initially asssume that the texts defy the 'hermeneutic code' of narrative (Cohan and Shires 1988: 123), which concerns the use of suspense as a structuring device. None the less, there *is* a compulsion in the narratives; we still want to know what happens next and how the story will unfold. To a considerable extent, this urgency of narrative force is constructed by the dramatic use of the present tense, so that there is an overlay of the 'true' present time from which the writer speaks, with the dramatic present in which significant moments are articulated. Perhaps this is to do, in part, with the omnipresent currency of living with cancer, as Julien suggests: 'Any cancer, once announced and then confirmed, carries on being described in the present – I have cancer – even when the cancerous tumour has been removed' (1996: 78). Benstock's characterization of a more traditional autobiographical genre may help to illustrate the distinctiveness of these texts in this respect: 'the Subject is made an Object of investiga-tion ... and is further divided between the present moment of narration and the past on which the narration is focused. These gaps in the temporal and spatial dimensions of the text are often success-fully hidden from reader and writer ... this view of the life history is grounded in authority' (Benstock 1998: 19). While her conclusion, that the self in women's autobiography is decentred or absent, is, as I hope I have shown, not valid in relation to these texts, there are crit-ical differences in narrative form and structuring which do mark an important shift from the traditional form of the genre.

The use of the present continuous tense is particularly significant in this respect; it implies an openness and a contingency of events (in contrast to the sense of authority which Benstock (1988) identifies in the traditional narrative form of autobiography), and an immediacy of connection with the reader. Characteristically, having closed her first chapter on an objective and generalized explanation of the process of biopsy, Mayer opens her second thus: the reader turns the page to an epigraphic quotation from Emily Dickinson, and then, 'An inch from my eyes, the expanse of fabric crosses my vision as far as I can see ... Above me somewhere, the great eye of the light is shining. A radio plays classical music. I am cold, lying naked under the thin cotton sheets and blanket with my bare buttocks against the greased metal grounding plate' (1993: 14). The juxtapositioning of the two tones is startling and disturbing, and exposes starkly just the kind of 'gap' in textual dimension that Benstock (1988: 18) claims is hidden in the traditional, masculine autobiographical narrative. The reader is drawn into the vivid trauma of the moment, the detail of the sensation described as though it were experienced now, with no sense of it being constructed as a remembered event; the Subject is of that moment, no 'Object of investigation' (*ibid.*). The episode recounted here is the return to consciousness after surgery; a similar immediacy is recovered in the narrative at other moments of dramatic intensity in Mayer's and others' stories.

Not all the texts, however, use this device of a shift of tense: Walder's (1992) narrative is exclusively in the present, while Colbourn's short essay (1996: 115–32) remains emphatically in the past. The effect of this latter text is of a completed discrete episode that is not to be seen to impinge on the present. (Interestingly, it is Colbourn, a GP, alone of these authors who expresses reservations about the reception of her story: 'it still alarms me that sometimes other people feel free to share my story' (*ibid.*: 122)). Dale's story (1996: 135-62) also remains resolutely and coherently in the past; her narrative is well ordered and linearly constructed, affirming a clear progression of events that reflects perhaps her final statement, describing her relation to her cancer, 'We try to hide from each other' (*ibid.*: 162). Her narrative uses a different device to keep a vital sense of the hermeneutic code. When she first locates the lump in her breast, 'Instinctively I knew at once that I had cancer' (*ibid.*: 137) and the reader knows this too, of course; the six months of denial, shock and numbness that intervene before a confirmed medical diagnosis provoke a narrative tension that defies any sense of temporal disloca-tion or authority. Acker's use of dramatized conversation serves a similar purpose (1997: 14), drawing the reader into the text as though it were a play staged before us, as though it were happening now. Lorde uses her diaries to inform her published narrative construction, so that past events are brought into an active present. This has the effect not of relegating her previous self to the status of an Object for study, as it might in clumsier hands, but of establishing a referential continuity between the times of writing, and between the states of identity. Butler and Rosenblum (1994) use this device too. Significantly, it is these three texts which most explicitly look to help others as well as themselves to make sense of their experience. The personal is brought to the fore in a rawer and less refined state, perhaps with the belief that closeness to the material will permit a beneficial or supportive proximity of writer and reader. But these texts also permit a gap for reflection, outside the temporal location of the events described. Cole's (1995) and Segrave's (1995) narratives, on the other hand, offer no refinement of the raw experience at all. They draw the reader into the diary account itself, leaving little space for reflection or analysis, and little potential for anything other than the present continuous involvement in the progression of the life/disease.

There is no selection of crucial 'moments of being', to use Virginia Woolf's term, and so no breathing space granted the reader.

The narrative coherence of all these texts is achieved through compliance with a formulaic patterning of structure – what can usefully be defined as the 'proairetic code' (Cohan and Shires 1998: 119). All are shaped by reference to several common and pivotal moments in the story: discovery, diagnosis, decisions about treatment, confronting possible death and life after treatment. So there is a chronologically linear narrative in the texts, a sense of being driven through the events – which perhaps reflects the ways in which the women's lives are presented as now driven by the disease: a relentless progression, a story unfolding. Lynch's book starts from the moment of discovery, so that the moment of epiphany is fixed to shape the ensuing narrative: 'I am stunned. Right under my fingers, as big as a wad of bubble gum, only harder, like the cap on the toothpaste tube. I feel it again, and my stomach jumps right up into my chest' (Lynch and Richards 1986: 5). Diagnosis, or 'the news', as Dale (1996) calls it, serves similarly in these texts as a central narrative point of focus. This ordering of the narrative through recounting significant events in the story of woman herself, of her interaction with the disease, the relationship between her and the disease, of her own psychic/spiritual development and growth, confers order, causality and meaningfulness, as Stanley (1992) has suggested.

Many of these narratives, however, deny the reader the sense of closure that the proairetic code suggests; the prescribed linear form that is the rational and coherent progression of the telling of a life is disrupted by the story of the cancer. The writer herself may well not know the end-point of the trajectory of the narrative as it has been plotted in the text; she does not know whether she will 'survive'. Her narrative may in fact not have an ending – several of these texts are completed by someone else (*viz.* Lynch and Richards 1986; Butler and Rosenblum 1994). The texts are left open in this way, and in each of them some sort of narrative device has to be adopted in order to make the text 'work', to impose a textual coherence. Frequently, this is a sense of the culmination of a particular episode, or some marker in the lifestory which is a marker to a new time. And, perhaps more interestingly, the very process of finishing the task of writing is a significant event in itself (as ever!); in this context it provides a distancing from the narrative of the disease, from the story that has occupied the pages. This may be marked by a shift in tense, or by a summing up of the events described in relation to the present. Several texts conclude with an account of how the woman has changed as a result of the story she has lived/told. Nkweto Simmonds, for example, lists the ways in which her life is different because of her experience of breast cancer (1996: 50-1). Her narrative closes, therefore, with a depiction of her as new self; she is not the same as the woman whose story is told in the preceding pages.

Selves and Identities

'Illness (is) the ultimate crisis of self-representation'.
                                                    (Spence 1995: 146)

In the process of these narratives, the disease, breast cancer itself, is shown to be not merely another predicate of the situated self, but to have a discrete identity in its own right, animated within the narratives. Thus Walder writes: 'The surgeon took it [the tumour] out using a local, and when he was done, I asked to see it ... It rested in the middle of a larger ball of pink and white breast tissue, sliced down the center like a hard-boiled egg, an onion-like layering of whitish-gray tissue about it, and I looked at it hard, trying to figure it out. We did not know it was cancer until twenty minutes later ... and then I was especially glad I had looked. Mano a mano, eyeball to eyeball' (1992: 1). Despite a mistaken conflation of the tumour – a symptom, with the cancer – a disease, this is a clear demonstration of how the narrative positions breast cancer as a central and separate protagonist. Initially, the tumour lies in the dish, an object of Walder's and the surgeon's gaze; by the time it is defined as a cancer, it has become animated and capable of returning that gaze – 'eyeball to eyeball'. In Dale's narrative (1996: 162), the cancer is animated as an active subject: 'It has become my stalker. I watch it over my shoulder'. In Julien's narrative, it becomes difficult to disentangle the multiplicity of positions which the woman with cancer occupies, and the referentiality of the various pronouns, but the cancer itself has a clearer identity: 'And so cancer, my contracted and concealed cancer, has developed its own language, an anti-language, a nocturnal writing ... ' (1996: 67). The texts establish an epistemological opposition between the woman and the disease, and this in turn allows for a parallel narrativization within the texts: the story of the woman and the story of the breast/cancer: '... "a cancer in your right breast." Did he say it twice or did I hear it twice? As he says it I feel my right breast detach itself from the rest of my body. It is no longer part of me' (Nkweto Simmonds 1996: 46). Brohn, however, from within a discourse of alternative medicine which may paradoxically encourage people with cancer to conceptualze themselves as separate from the disease for healing purposes, insists that 'my cancer involved the whole of me, not just a bumpy bit on the left hand side going down' (Brohn 1987: 4). But this does not preclude the elevation of the disease to the status of an animated identity in her text, nor in Cole's, who talks directly to her tumour from within a similar discursive position: '"Hi! Lump, I know you're there and I don't mind, providing you don't go walkabout. Keep calm and peaceful and relax"' (Cole 1995: 378).

Other identities are revealed in the texts too, and new ones emerge. While it is widely accepted as a truism in all sorts of contemporary discourses that we are changed by life-threatening events, the new sense of self is not *necessarily* either outside or prior, nor more authentic, than the alternative or previous identities. The texts bring together all the different selves around the unfolding of the story of the disease: before and after diagnosis and treatment, and reveal the lines of demarcation and fracture. Spence writes of 'the separation of disciplines, of split identities – in this case, me as "cancer patient" without any history except a medical one, versus me as "artist" rendered unproductive through illness' (Spence 1995: 130).

The starting point for the recognition of the different selves is frequently the alienation and sense of the *loss* of self that diagnosis and treatment of breast cancer provoke. Thus the story itself may reveal the discrete strands. This is powerfully emphasized in Lynch's accounts of the questioning she received as she went in for a biopsy: '"Are you Dorothea? ... Hello, are you Dorothea? ... Are you Dorothea Lynch?"', and the same when she awakes from surgery (Lynch and Richards 1986: 11 and 290), reinforcing her own sense of dislocation. Later she recounts how 'I don't even feel like the same person' (*ibid.*: 60) since the operation. Richards' photographs illustrate this transformation, recording the differences in her private and public appearance. A personal and textual clash of discourse or of reality may initially engender a movement away from the 'old' and towards a 'new' structuring of self-identity: a confrontation with a physician or unhappiness with what is offered by way of treatment. Brohn writes, 'A role was being forced on me that I simply could not and would not bear' (Brohn 1987: 54). Similarly, Acker says of the surgical procedures she endured: 'I was being reduced to something I couldn't recognize' (Acker, 1997: 14).

All the texts demonstrate 'the processes and structures of identification – both psychic and social', not that the 'subject simply "has" an
identity' (Ahmed 1997: 157). The narratives call the writers to a
variety of subject positions, alongside and against the past selves, the
'master narratives' of cancer and their own bodily experiences. Often
it is through the body that these new subjectivities and new resis-
tances (in the Foucauldian sense) are realized. The body and the
identity of the woman with breast cancer become contested sites of
meaning between the hegemony of the discourse of medical practice
and her own sense of the disease and her relationship to it, the
meaning she generates through the process. The self, as Braidotti has
shown, is 'anchored in this living matter ... a layer of corporeal materiality' (Braidotti 1994: 165), and so the 'core self' incorporates these
inner and outer changes.

Audre Lorde's renowned decision not to wear a prosthesis offers
valuable insights into her perception of the relationship between the
old and the changed selves.

> To imply to a woman that yes, she can be the 'same' as before
> surgery, with the skillful application of a little puff of lambswool,
> and/or silicone gel, is to place an emphasis upon prosthesis which
> encourages her not to deal with herself as physically and emotion-
> ally real, even though altered and traumatised ... With quick
> cosmetic reassurance, we are told ... our appearance is all, the sum
> total of self. I did not have to look down at the bandages on my
> chest to know that I did not feel the same as before surgery. But I
> still felt like myself, like Audre ... (Lorde 1980: 57)

Both recognition of change and a continuity of self are implied
here, an uncomfortable tension that other women recount too. And as
Kelly and Field (1996: 248), point out, perhaps stating the obvious, 'As
an individual moves from situation to situation, as their body changes
and as their illness develops, there is still an important sense in which
they are the same person they were before their body began to alter,
albeit in a different social situation'. But against the two models they
suggest, these texts demonstrate that illness/breast cancer is neither
simply about 'identity change' (the 'crisis approach'), nor a 'process of
loss of self' (the 'negotiation model'). Rather, what is revealed is the
layering of identity, an accretion, each recognizable to a 'core' self.
Thus Mayer's breast reconstruction comes, as she recognizes, 'to have
a much larger symbolic meaning ... the reconstructed breast retained

its power as a metaphor for my whole sense of self, but the symbol was becoming increasingly mixed. I was the same person – sort of, until you looked closely – but my inner landscape had radically changed' (1993: 114). She admits to sharing Lorde's views, and somehow to having hoped the surgery might restore her former self; and, further, she agrees with Lorde: 'I knew exactly what she meant. It was this precise discrepancy that had caused me so much anguish, trying to reconcile the gap between what I felt and how I looked', and to her 'disappointments with reconstruction ... [being] more with how it felt to incorporate this "stranger" into my body' (*ibid.*). As she also acknowledges, this state of dissatisfaction with her body is felt by many Western women, is common enough.

The texts, then, offer a series of fragments, an accretion of selves accompanied by some erosion too. And so the narrative construction of these multiple identities reveals the inappropriateness and inexactitude of an essentialist notion of the self, defined by Fuss as 'most commonly understood as a belief in the real true essence of things, the invariable and fixed properties which define the "whatness" of a given entity' (Fuss 1989: xi). The subject of the texts is a 'subject in process', her identities 'constantly called into question, brought to trial, overruled' (Kristeva 1996: 351). As Mayer says (1993: 59), 'I was, in a sense, moving from one identity to another. The change from student writer to cancer patient seemed merely another kind of graduation to a new and more demanding post-graduate level of study'. Fuss shows how postmodernism claims two alternative theories of the self; the false, unitary and essentialist self, or an equally undifferentiated but totally historically or textually constituted 'true' one (Fuss 1989: 210). She suggests that women's experience, however, can help elucidate a difference between a core self and the essentialist self: stressing the importance of social relations in self-formation. This seems to be true not just of early influences in a life, as she suggests, but of the endless stream of interaction with the world which living entails, and of the many shifts in social situations, dramatically emphasized by life-threatening illness.

Writing the Self

Benstock states, however, that there remains always a 'gap that the drive toward unity of self can never entirely close' (Benstock 1998: 12). Certainly some of these texts can conform to a dominant theme within 'alternative' medical discourse, by which, as Stacey points out:

'With the correct guidance, the cancer patient can discover a new self, a true self, an Ur-self (or original self); you are invited to "become who you are", or rather, to become "who you should have been"' (1996: 12). Spence (1995: 135) aims to 'confront the neurotically induced notion of an idealized self' through her stories of disease and illness, presenting instead the fragmented parts of her identity. The 'original' self, the 'unified' or 'idealized' self, sound like Fuss's 'essentialist' self, an *a priori* authentic being hovering intangible and elusive, but assumed to be omnipresent. Nowhere, however, is it/she apparent in the texts. Of greater import is the relationship between these identities imposed by the texts *qua* text: a published and discrete entity that manifestly holds together those selves, 'the multiplicity of split-off fragments which go to make up an apparently coherent identity' (Spence 1995: 135). So the gap is not closed: the discrete parts remain evident, but they are held in connection by the narrative itself. As Friedman suggests, alienation 'from the historically imposed image of the self is what motivates the writing, the creation of an alternate self in the autobiographical act' (Friedman 1998: 41). But, crucially, we are asked to believe in the referential 'truth' of these accounts, of real women in a real world – quite against the Lacanian and poststructuralist concepts of the self which maintain it is a fictive entity.

We have already seen how the act of writing constructs meaningfulness; the construction of the self, a changed self, is articulated through the same processes. Telling stories is how we make ourselves – in a whole range of ways, which Stacey (1996: 12) illustrates. 'Language is the medium by and through which the "self" is constructed', as Benstock (1998: 29) tells us. Thus here we can see how writing a lifestory becomes the construction of a new identity, a literal inscribing of the self, and publication the means by which that new identity is to be recognized, known and legitimated. As Trinh T. Minh-ha has it: 'To write is to become. Not to become a writer (or a poet), but to become, intransitively' (Minh-ha 1989: 19). This is the public and political significance of women writing their lives, 'taking the power of words, of representation, into their own hands' (Friedman 1998: 40), and is related to an earlier observation that the writers position themselves as subjects within a liberal humanist tradition, asserting the identity of the self, as rational, responsible and self-conscious. It remains an important project for women with breast cancer whose experience too readily constructs them as 'subjected being(s)', who are required still to 'submit to the authority of social formation' (Eagleton 1996: 340). The subject is understood in these texts through a process of becoming, rather than of being.

Reflecting on a conversation with her surgeon, Acker tells how 'conventional medicine was reducing me, quickly, to a body that was only material, to a body without hope and so without will, to a puppet who, separated by fear from her imagination and vision, would do whatever she was told' (1997: 14). It is against how she is constructed here as a subjected subject, that she determines to assert her own sense of self: 'Did I have anything in myself, in my life, that could help me know and so deal with cancer? My answer was: it takes strength to know. Where then is my strength? Answer: in my work, my writing' (*ibid.:* 21). Both Acker and Spence write their stories of breast cancer against the generalization posited by Ahmed, that: 'Auto-biography may write its subject only insofar as it renders its subject a subject, that is, an embodied and located entity which is representable only through its partial negation or loss' (Ahmed 1997: 154).

If illness leads, as Turner (1984: 235) suggests, to a devaluation of the self, then the work of these narratives, and the engagement with breast cancer, may be seen to involve the revaluation of the self. From a symbolic interactionist perspective, he observes that illness under-mines the coherence of personal identity and is a negation of self-concept. These narratives explicitly concern processes of reap-praisal and the construction or emergence of new identities, through active agency. Stacey (1998) has shown how this process sits firmly within a romantic literary tradition, but the texts importantly offer more than that, and are positioned within a politically purposeful genre which includes 'coming out stories'. Thus Stanley's study of published accounts of coming out usefully informs an understanding of the narrative structuring and thematic emphases in these breast cancer texts too: these autobiographies also 'centralise self-alienation, lack of self-knowledge and coherence ... [and] see the emergent more authentic self as beset by the negative reactions of others ... [They] are concerned with achieving a greater degree of self-authenticity ... ' Furthermore, they 'also have considerable ontological and epistemo-logical consequence, for the entire nature of 'reality' and one's relationship to it is thereby changed' (Stanley 1992: 117–18). The similarities with Turner's thesis of the social effects of illness are very evident in this analysis, but it is *against* these effects that these narra-tives are constructed. As Mayer says, she writes 'to form a new image, a new sense of who I am' (1993: 6), and to position herself anew against the 'experience of alienation from the normal, healthy world' (*ibid.*: 30).

Cole's story illustrates this process too. The focus on self-construction, on becoming her authentic self, is so emphatic that the other participants in her narrative are seldom directly reported and remain unanimated within the text; all dialogue and interaction is mediated through her own consciousness and commentary. One of the effects of this, within the text, is to create two Jenny Coles: the one to whom these events happen and the other commenting sardonically and in expletives from the sidelines. And there is a third too, the woman she believes the medics see in their treatment of her, who is so often referred to as 'Mrs Cole' – to her irritation; being called by her name – Jenny – becomes an important signifier of how she wants to be known, to herself and to the world (Cole 1995: 120). Her text is also constructed as dialogue between these different selves; 'she' talks to or at 'herself' (*ibid*.: 316). Wilber's account of his wife's experience of breast cancer, which is derived in large part from her journals, describes how she, Terry, marked her fortieth birthday by changing her name. She decided to redefine herself in a less masculine way and to reject the aspects of her life and work which she regarded as having always been masculinized. She told all her friends that she was now Treya, a more feminine name, short for Estrella (Wilber 1991). This 'demand for recognition and for the restoration of identity through language, through the authority of proper names' (Felman 1989: 149) marks very clearly the shift to a new self. The public articulation of this identity makes the process akin to the coming out to friends and family recounted in the texts Stanley studied, and distinguishes it from the unwonted impositioning and renegotiating of social identity that illness inevitably provokes anyway (Kelly and Field 1996).

Other identities are revealed differently in the narratives; in recognizing the proairetic codification of the texts, a pivotal moment describes the writer looking in a mirror at her new, post-surgery self. This directly invokes Lacan's work on psychic development and the way in which the 'mirror stage' 'serves up a false image of the child's unified "self". This unity is imposed from the outside ... [and] must, therefore, be understood as a metaphor for the vision of harmony of a subject essentially in discord' (Benstock 1998: 12). In these texts, however, the writers all recount a sense of dispersion of the self, a recognition that the reflection is a distortion, a dislocation from previous selves, and certainly that there is no immediate acceptance of the new identity they see. Dale says, 'I caught sight of my reflection in the mirror as I stepped into the bath. Suddenly I was filled with self-loathing and a sense of self-betrayal' (Dale 1996: 159). Lynch, who in common with other women, found the loss of her hair following chemotherapy to represent a particularly potent loss of a past self, describes looking in her bathroom mirror: 'Bald; lashless, eyebrowless; scaly patches of red, dry skin all over my face; thick blackened scar tissue where my breast once was. I am dried up, older than ancient, sexless. My body is unfamiliar territory to me' (Lynch and Richards 1986: 58). The photographs Richards takes of her, for them both, also record this changing identity, and serve as permanent records of the new reflections. And Mayer writes: 'I kept on staring at myself, trying to come to terms with this newly lopsided person staring back at me from the mirror', revealing to her 'how profoundly and permanently I'd been changed' (1993: 38).

A 'vision of harmony', an integration of these disparate identities and selves, becomes the task of the writing, even though there may be no sense of unifying these selves, through mirror-reflection, or through the narrative construction. It may be accomplished by the sense in some of the texts of a continuity between what Benstock refers to as the I-then and the I-now. So Lorde writes in her journal, 'I looked at the large gentle curve my left breast made under the pajama top, a curve that seemed even larger now that it stood by itself. I looked strange and uneven and peculiar to myself, but somehow, ever so much more myself … and either I would love my body one-breasted now, or remain forever alien to myself' (Lorde 1980: 44). And Julien too: 'This morning, in the mirror, *I looked at myself,* for a long time, aware of the conventions of this face to face, but determined to persist. In fact, the two of us were summoned. In answering this summons, something had to happen between us, standing there … A harmony began to show itself on our withered skin' (Julien 1996: 92). Scars and disfigurements are cultural inscriptions on the body; they challenge our internalized sense of the valorization of wholeness and symmetry as concomitant with beauty. Creating any continuity, integrity, of selves against this cultural alienation from bodily identity radically repositions these women with breast cancer against what Rowbotham describes as 'the distorting identities imposed by culture'. As she says, women have 'left "the sign" of their "presence" in their autobiographical writings' (Friedman 1988: 56); that sign is inscribed by the narratives themselves, and establishes a quite new, discrete and integrated identity to the narrators.

Against what she calls the 'wipe-out of self in which women are constantly encouraged to take part', Lorde (1980: 64), asserts the need for women with mastectomies to 'become visible to each other', as a first step which will 'translate the silence surrounding breast cancer into language and action against this scourge' (*ibid.*: 61). That visibility, she claims, also provides mutual support, and her writing is one way in which she seeks to promote that. The creation of new identities within these narratives is constructed by an act of writing that leads beyond the sense of alienation, of disgust, horror, fear and of mutilation provoked by looking in the mirror. So these autobiographical narratives, already identified as in many respects being a shared endeavour, are an expression of Rowbotham's statement that 'women can move beyond alienation through a collective solidarity with other women', and 'project [their] own image onto history' (Friedman 1988: 40).

Finally, then, this is the important project of these texts. The verbalization, the publication, of personal narratives of breast cancer place these women centre-stage, and place breast cancer there too, for, as we have seen, breast cancer is a crucial subjectivity within the texts in its own right. These are not 'spotlight' autobiographies, to use Stanley's (1992) term; the authors are not 'important' public figures, but they acquire authority, and their stories become 'valorized accounts' (*ibid.*), through the process of writing and of publication. The variety of the narratives reveals the diversity of individual experience, while the commonality of experience emphasizes the political import of breast cancer, which 'we cannot afford to ... consider ... as a private nor secret personal problem' (Lorde 1980: 61). What the narratives also demonstrate are the processes by which the narrators come to position themselves in relation to a new subject position, as a 'woman with breast cancer'. Not as a victim, a survivor or a sufferer, although each of those subjectivities may also be self-ascribed too, but as a self carrying that new position within her; a position made public and political by the process of 'coming out' as such, and by publishing her account.

The subjects are not, however, fixed by this process, nor is 'woman with breast cancer' an ontologically discrete category. The new subjectivity does not replace previous subject positions, as I have shown; it is not a 'singular name' (Ahmed 1997: 155); not a 'unitary, self-directed, isolated ego' (Waugh 1996: 360). Braidotti's distinction between identity and subjectivity is useful to illustrate the distinctiveness of this process of becoming, not being, and what I believe is ultimately the truly revolutionary nature of these texts: 'Identity bears a privileged bond to the unconscious processes, whereas political subjectivity is a conscious and willed position' (Braidotti 1994: 166).

So while the narratives recount the layers of self-identity crucial to the narrator's own lifestory, there is this further subjectivity defined by a positioning in the world, as shared and collective, and in opposition to the 'master narratives' of what it is to be a woman and to have breast cancer. As Butler (1990: 142) states, 'the "doer" is invariably constructed in and through the deed' – in this case, through the act of living with the breast cancer.

Just as Wittig's (1992) lesbian 'carries the straight woman within us', so the 'woman with breast cancer' carries her previous selves, her undiseased self, her future self, within her too, as the telling of her story shows. There are varying degrees of harmonization between these subjectivities, but in each she emerges as a self visible to herself and to her reading public. From the process of transformation of which Lorde writes, through the act of speaking or writing out, emerges a revolutionary new figure, in collective solidarity with those other 'women with breast cancer': the 'warriors' in Lorde's phrase (Lorde 1980: 60). As such, she has the status of Wittig's lesbian, Haraway's cyborg and Moraga's mestiza – grouped together in this illuminating way by Eagleton (1996: 347): women positioned on the margins of given identities, asserting the power of naming their defining experience. The location of these 'warriors' on the Borderlands (Anzaldua 1987) is determined by their experience of breast cancer; while a collective subjectivity as woman-with-breast-cancer defines one subject position, it is not, as I have shown, the whole story. 'The new *mestiza* copes by developing a tolerance for contradictions, a tolerance for ambiguity' (*ibid.*: 79), and the woman-with-breast-cancer survives in just such a state of uncertainty, in flux. Rowbotham claims that

> In order to create an alternative an oppressed group must at once shatter the self-reflecting world which encircles it and, at the same time, project its own image onto history. In order to discover its own identity as distinct from that of the oppressor it has to be visible to itself. People who are without names, who do not know themselves ... experience a kind of paralysis of consciousness. The first step is to connect ... (1973: 27–9)

This, then, is the process of publishing the personal, establishing identity through the process of narrativization of a lifestory, these stories of breast cancer, which make the writers visible in their own image.

Note

1 (I grant that this perhaps is testament to my own generally positive experience of c.r., and that other women's experiences may not indicate this at all; none the less, this was the expressed political *purpose* of the process, and that position may be used with some validity, I think.

References

The Autobiographical Stories

Acker, K. 'The Gift of Disease', *The Guardian* (18 January 1997).
Batt, S. *Patient No More: The Politics of Breast Cancer* (London: Scarlet Press 1994).
Brohn, P. *Gentle Giants* (London: Century Hutchinson 1987).
Butler, S. and B. Rosenblum, *Cancer in Two Voices* (London: The Women's Press 1994).
Colbourn, C. 'Refugees in a Strange Country'. In Duncker, P. and V. Wilson eds. *Cancer: Through the Eyes of Ten Women* (London: Pandora 1996).
Cole, J. *Journey (with a Cancer)* (London: Pawprints 1995).
Dale, E. 'The Lump' in Duncker, P. and V. Wilson, eds. *Cancer: Through the Eyes of Ten Women* (London: Pandora 1996).
Julien, J. 'Sweat' in Duncker, P. and V. Wilson, eds. *Cancer: Through the Eyes of Ten Women* (London: Pandora 1996).
Lorde, A. *The Cancer Journals* (San Francisco: Spinsters Ink 1980).
Lynch, D. and E. Richards *Exploding into Life* (New York: Aperture 1986).
Mayer, M. *Examining Myself: One Woman's Story of Breast Cancer Treatment and Recovery* (Boston: Faber and Faber 1993).
Nkweto Simmonds, F. 'A Remembering' in eds. Duncker, P. and V. Wilson.
Rosenblum, B. '"I Have Begun the Process of Dying"' in Spence, J. and P. Holland, eds., *Family Snaps: The Meanings of Domestic Photography* (London: Virago 1991).
Segrave, E. *The Diary of a Breast* (London: Faber and Faber 1997).
Spence, J. *Cultural Sniping: The Art of Transgression* (London: Routledge, 1995).
Stacey, J. 'Conquering Heroes: The Politics of Cancer Narratives' in eds. Duncker, P. and V. Wilson.
Walder, J. *My Breast: One Woman's Story* (London: The Women's Press 1994).
Wilber, K. *Grace and Grit: The Life and Death of Treya Killam Wilber* (Boston: Shambhala 1991)

Other Sources

Ahmed, S. '"It's a Sun-tan, Isn't it?': Auto-biography as an Identificatory Practice'. In Mirza, H.S., ed. *Black British Feminism* (London: Routledge 1997).
Anzaldua, G. *Borderlands/La Frontera: The New Mestiza* (San Francisco: Spinsters, Aunt Lute 1990).
Benstock, S. *The Private Self: The Theory and Practice of Women's Autobiographical Writings* (Chapel Hill, NC and London: University of North Carolina Press 1988).
Braidotti, R. *Nomadic Subjects. Embodiment and Sexual Difference in Contemporary*

Feminist Theory (New York and Chichester, West Sussex: Columbia University Press 1994).

Brodski, B. and C. Schenk, eds. *Life/Lives: Theorizing Women's Autobiography* (Ithaca, NY: Cornell University Press 1988).

Butler, J. *Gender Trouble: Feminism and the Subversion of Identity* (London: Routledge 1990).

Cartwright, L. 'Community and the Public Body in Breast Cancer Media Activism', *Cultural Studies* 12(2) (1998) pp. 117–38.

Cixous, H. 'Sorties: Out and Out: Attacks/Ways Out/Forays' in Belsey, C. and J. Moore, eds. *The Feminist Reader: Essays in Gender and The Politics of Literary Criticism* (London: Macmillan 1989).

Cohan, S. and L.M. Shires. *Telling Stories. A Theoretical Analysis of Narrative Fiction* (London: Routledge 1988).

Culler, J. *The Pursuit of Signs: Semiotics, Literature, Deconstruction* (London: Routledge and Kegan Paul 1981).

Duncker, P. *Sisters and Strangers: An Introduction to Contemporary Feminist Fiction* (London: Blackwell 1992).

Felman, S. 'Women and Madness: the Critical Phallacy'. In Belsey, C. and J. Moore, eds. *The Feminist Reader* (London: Macmillan 1989).

Flax, J. *Thinking Fragments* (Berkeley: University of California Press 1990).

Friedman, S.S. 'Women's Auto-Biographical Selves: Theory and Practice'. In Benstock, S. *The Private Self* (Chapel Hill, NC and London: University of North Carolina Press 1988).

Fuss, D. *Essentially Speaking: Feminism, Nature and Difference* (London: Routledge 1989).

Haraway, D. 'A Manifesto for Cyborgs: Science, Technology and Socialist Feminism in the 1980s' in Nicholson, L. ed. *Feminism/Postmodernism* (London: Routledge 1990).

Jelinek, E. *Women's Autobiography: Essays in Criticism* (Bloomington: Indiana University Press 1980).

Joolz (in performance, York, Spring 1997).

Juhasz, S. 'Toward a Theory of Form in Feminist Autobiography: Kate Millett's *Flying* and *Sita;* Maxine Hong Kingston's *The Woman Warrior'*, in Jelinek, E., ed. *Women's Autobiography: Essays in Criticism* (Bloomington: Indiana University Press 1980).

Kearney, R. *The End of the Story?* (BBC Radio 3, 4 October 1996).

Kelly, M.P. and D. Field, 'Medical Sociology, Chronic Illness and the Body', *Sociology of Health and Illness* Vol.18, No.2 (1996) pp. 241–57.

Kristeva, J. 'A Question of Subjectivity: An Interview', in Eagleton, M. *Feminist Literary Theory, A Reader* (Oxford: Blackwell 1996).

Lury, C. 'The Difference in Women's Writing: Essays on the Rise of Personal Experience', *Studies in Sexual Politics* (Manchester University 1987).

McRobbie, A. 'Feminism, Postmodernism and the Real Me'. In Perryman, M., ed., *Altered States: Postmodernism, Politics, Culture* (London: Lawrence and Wishart 1994).

Rowbotham, S. *Women's Consciousness, Man's World* (London: Penguin 1973).

Said, E.W. *Orientalism* (Harmondsworth: Penguin 1995).

Shildrick, M. *Leaky Bodies and Boundaries. Feminism, Postmodernism and (Bio)ethics* (London: Routledge 1997).

Sontag, S. *Illness as Metaphor* (Harmondsworth: Penguin 1979).

Stacey, J. *Teratologies, A Cultural Study of Cancer* (London: Routledge 1997).

Stanley, L. *The Auto/biographical I: The Theory and Practice of Feminist Auto/biography* (Manchester: Manchester University Press 1992).

Trinh T., Minh-ha. *Woman, Native, Other: Writing Postcoloniality and Feminism* (Bloomington and Indianapolis: Indiana State University 1989).

Turner, B. *The Body and Society: Explorations in Social Theory* (Oxford: Blackwell 1984).

Waugh, P. 'Feminine Fictions: Revisiting the Postmodern'. In Eagleton, M. *Feminist Literary Theory, A Reader* (Oxford: Blackwell 1996).

Wittig, M. *The Straight Mind and Other Essays* (Hemel Hempstead: Harvester Wheatsheaf 1992).

Yardley, L. *Material Discourses of Health and Illness* (London: Routledge 1997).

Yorke, L. *Adrienne Rich: Passion, Politics and the Body* (London: Sage 1997).

Part II

Discourses of Risk and Breast Cancer

5
Controversies in Breast Cancer Prevention: the Discourse of Risk[1]

Christy Simpson

'Risk' is probably one of the most familiar and commonly used terms in discussions about breast cancer prevention. Women, doctors, government officials and others talk about whether someone is at either a high or low risk of developing this disease, how the risk of getting breast cancer can be reduced, and what the risks of certain forms of prevention are. Risk is a word that typically connotes fear or anxiety, implying that someone is, in a sense, in danger; many women are concerned about their risk of developing breast cancer and make medical decisions based upon their perceived risk(s). Further, there is controversy about the current strategies being investigated for breast cancer prevention, such as prophylactic mastectomy and tamoxifen; the latter of which will be discussed below. In this chapter, I will examine how the discussion of, focus on and attention to breast cancer risk connects to different ideologies about health and disease, and, in particular, how these ideologies shape the strategies pursued for breast cancer prevention. A better understanding of risk discourse will greatly enhance this investigation into the role of ideology in breast cancer prevention. For my purposes, an ideology is understood to be a system or collection of values and beliefs, especially those concerning social or political matters, held by an individual or group (Webster's Ninth New Collegiate Dictionary 1989; Martin 1994).

There are many different ways of thinking about risk or framing a discussion about risk; for example, taking a psychological or sociological perspective. In the following, I will describe a philosophical approach to risk I wish to take. This approach will allow me to identify and critically evaluate the ideological underpinnings of breast cancer prevention risk discourse, and yield my conclusion that, ideologically speaking, a pluralistic approach to risk and the prevention of breast cancer is necessary.

The Conceptual Framework

Risk Assessment

The first step in generating this philosophical approach to risk is to acknowledge that there are at least three different levels at which breast cancer risk discourse is primarily conducted. These are: (1) the level of individual women who are concerned about their risk of developing breast cancer and who want to know what they can do to prevent or avoid getting this disease;[2] (2) the level of science and the research agenda set both for investigating risk and for discovering methods to decrease or prevent certain risks; and (3) the societal level where there exists a variety of socio-political aims and a plurality of values, each potentially affecting the relative ranking of which strategies for the prevention of breast cancer will be promoted or funded. In other words, discussion about risk can occur at each of the personal, scientific and social levels. Data generated about risk by the scientific community will necessarily affect what information both individuals and society have about risk and its application to decision-making about possible risk-reducing measures. Further, the scientific level of risk discourse and assessment can be affected in many ways by the interests of both individuals and society; for example, as a result of (political) pressure applied by a group of individuals, it is possible that the research agenda for breast cancer prevention may shift. It should be emphasized that individuals often perceive risk differently from the way science does and this difference is one source of conflict between the identified levels of risk discourse. Thus, it becomes clear that, although there are at least three discrete levels at which risk discourse commonly takes place, there is much communication and interplay between these levels; the risk discourse at one level can have an effect on the risk discourse at another.

Much of the recent research and thought on risk and risk assessment has tried to unravel the different factors that come into play when a decision about risk is made. One of the biggest shifts in thinking about risk has been the identification of the role of values and ideologies in risk discourse (Brunk 1991; Cranor 1990; Hansson 1993). No longer does the determination of risk via statistical methods enjoy its objective authority in discussions. As is now beginning to be demonstrated, value judgements and ideological commitments are an integral part of risk – a part that needs to be explored and made explicit if we (as individuals, as scientists, and as a society) are to comprehend more fully how 'risk' is calculated, communicated, perceived and accepted.

K.S. Shrader-Frechette (1991) offers an analysis of risk assessment that, in many ways, maps on to the three levels of risk discourse identified above and helps to provide a more complete description of the various facets of risk and its assessment. She breaks risk assessment down into three different parts, each of which has an important role in the overall analysis of risk at the individual, scientific and social levels. First, there is the choice of topics for risk assessment; that is, what should be looked at? What do we, for example, as individuals, *need* to know the risk of? What do we *want* to know the risk of? For each individual, depending on the circumstances and direction one's life takes, knowing about certain risks will be more important than knowing about others. For example, women who have a family history of early onset breast cancer will be more likely to want to know whether they carry the breast cancer genes and the attendant risks of developing this disease than women without this family history. In much the same way, setting the scientific research agenda or determining what safety measures should be instituted in our communities is affected by what is deemed to be important to know the risks of and/or what it is important to protect people from. Priorities about risks are set at each of the individual, scientific and social levels and this is where values and ideologies come in; ideological commitments help to determine and structure what these priorities will be.

Second, once an area of risk is chosen for investigation, information about this risk is frequently sought. Typically, scientific research is relied on to generate this information for individual, medical and societal use. As Shrader-Frechette points out, values and ideological commitments can and do affect even this part of risk assessment. Decisions must be made with respect to what data are relevant, if there are enough data, and which statistical tool(s) should be used; all of these decisions involve making methodological judgements about how the research will proceed. There are many gaps in scientific knowledge and how these gaps or uncertainties are dealt with relates very closely to what is believed to qualify as 'good' science or 'proper' procedure. Science cannot proceed without making certain assumptions or judgement calls, such as these. As I will discuss more fully below, the recognition of these types of value judgements in scientific discourse does not automatically entail that all the information science gives us is incorrect or completely biased. Shrader-Frechette emphasizes that awareness of these types of judgements and how they may affect or shape the data about risk can help individuals, policy-makers and others to assess the information. For example, in determining whether a certain chemical is carcinogenic, assumptions will have to made about the type (skin contact vs. ingestion), length (short vs. long term), and level (low vs. acute doses) of exposure. If it is decided that the most likely exposures to this chemical are acute, short-term, skin contact exposures, then the information generated with respect to the carcinogenic properties of this chemical will necessarily only apply in these types of situations; as such, it is essential that these types of judgements about exposures be acknowledged and available for consideration.

Third, and finally, having generated some data about the risk(s) in question, these data need to be evaluated – by society, by the scientific community and by individuals. These evaluations may be different or diverse in relation to the various ideological commitments that frame how the 'numbers' are understood and are used to make decisions. Various questions can be asked about the risk data: Is this risk minimal? Is this risk below acceptable standards? Is this a risk I/society needs to be concerned about? Should I/society do something about this risk? Can I/society alter this level of risk? Would more information about this risk be helpful? Do these data meet peer-reviewed standards in science? It is highly unlikely that decisions about risk can be made without the utilization of some value structure or ideology(ies) as these will provide the context in which the relevant data and information will be assessed. Values and ideologies are more commonly recognized as being involved in the evaluation of risk as this is where much of the controversy over risk and appropriate inter-ventions is typically found. For example, it may be decided at the social level (by the public health authorities) that a certain chemical with carcinogenic properties is safe for use as a pesticide, given that the risks of developing cancer are minimal when exposure to the chemical is low and that consumers would be only exposed to minute amounts of this chemical. In contrast, at the individual level, some consumers may decide not to eat vegetables exposed to this pesticide believing that even minute exposures to this carcinogenic chemical are too high.

By using Shrader-Frechette's breakdown of the three aspects of risk assessment in conjunction with the identified levels of risk discourse, it becomes apparent that the importance of values and ideological commitments and the role they play in risk discourse must be acknowledged. While there is much data available about breast cancer risk and a predictable increase of data in the future, none of these facts means anything if not placed within a context. These contexts will vary between individuals and societies and, consequently, controversies about risk can arise. In using the framework described above and by paying particular attention to the role of ideology(ies), the reasons for and motivations behind these controversies about risk can be identified and made sense of.

As part of this approach to risk, it needs to be emphasized that the involvement of ideologies in risk assessment and risk discourse does not mean that science is completely subjective and cannot provide *any* useful information (about risk). In fact, science gives us, as individuals and as a society, much information that has helped and will continue to help improve our lives, information that will make us healthier and information that will reduce disease. A number of technological and pharmacological measures have arisen from scientific research that have had positive effects on our lives. But there is still much to investigate and learn about. One of the outcomes of this ongoing research process is that there is not always enough information at a given time for definitive conclusions; as a result, science sometimes provides information about risk that is ambiguous. For example, a new treatment may not be clearly beneficial or harmful; that is, the information generated about the risks of the treatment can be evaluated in different ways and on some evaluations it may prove to be beneficial, while on others it will not. In other words, depending on what context the information is evaluated in, whether by the individual, by science or by society, and what ideological perspectives are applied, different evaluations of, or recommendations about, this treatment could be made. While science can set some constraints and close off certain possibilities (for example, it is known that penicillin will not have any effect on a viral infection), it can also leave 'open questions'. Judgements made with respect to these open questions will rely on values and ideologies. Later in this chapter, I will discuss chemoprevention measures for breast cancer, paying particular attention to tamoxifen. There is vigorous debate about tamoxifen in relation to its respective value and potential harms, that is, about the risks versus the benefits of taking this drug. The data generated thus far about tamoxifen can be categorized as ambiguous; the questions under investigation then are: How does the risk assessment of this drug proceed at the levels of individual women, science and society, and what effects do different ideologies have on this risk discourse?

Three Important Ideologies

This discussion needs to be contextualized in relation to three prominent ideological positions which can be identified in discussions of
health and disease. The first of these concerns the belief in technological and pharmacological solutions to problems of health and
disease – henceforth referred to as the technology ideology – and
points to the many successes of new technologies and pharmacologies
in curing individuals of disease and in helping to prevent disease.
While in many cases the use of new technology or a new drug will
help a number of persons, these options will also be found not to help
many others and may even do harm to some. Yet the large degree of
positive attention given to new medical breakthroughs within
contemporary culture makes it difficult to question or resist this technological push and to pursue other options for dealing with problems
of health and disease, such as reducing the number of carcinogens in
our environment. The dominant belief in the value and worthiness of
science helps to reinforce this ideology, at times with good reason, but
the interests of 'big business', that is, multinational companies, in
promoting this perspective cannot be ignored; the profit to be made
from new drugs and new technologies is very real.

The second ideological perspective of relevance here is the emphasis on the promotion of personal or individual responsibility for
health; this ideology suggests that it is up to each person to take
control of his/her health. The assumption is that if this is done properly and with commitment, most diseases or health problems will be
avoided. Personal responsibility for disease is typically presented in
terms of lifestyle choices, such as changing one's diet, exercising, quit-
ting smoking and pursuing opportunities for early detection and cure
of disease. And while it is true that these provisions can decrease one's
chances of getting a number of diseases, following these provisions
should not be taken to mean one will never get sick. The high profile
of the personal responsibility ideology (to the exclusion of consideration of other factors that play a role in determining health status, such
as the environment in which one lives) helps to reinforce the attitude
that disease or risk of disease is something experienced by individuals
and should therefore be addressed by individuals. This focus on individuals also promotes a short-term perspective on health and disease
as attention is directed towards educating and changing the behaviours of current individuals, a process that will have to be repeated for
each generation. Given this (over)emphasis on personal responsibil-

ity, it is understandable that many people are anxious about becoming sick if for no other reason than if they do become sick, the ideology of personal responsibility suggests that it may be because they were not vigilant enough in warding it off. In the case of breast cancer, with its media attention and the oft-repeated '1-in-9 lifetime risk of developing breast cancer', it is understandable that many women are scared about developing this disease. Thus, it becomes important to think about how information about risk, breast cancer and personal responsibility for this disease is presented in the media and how its framing can contribute to the fear women experience. Of course, individual women are and should be concerned about breast cancer (at least to some extent) and will want to do everything possible to avoid getting this disease, but the focus on personal responsibility for avoiding breast cancer should not obscure the risks created by, for example, living in a polluted environment and the need for social responsibility with respect to health and disease – a need that should and must be addressed by the social level of risk discourse.

The third dominant ideological discourse, the social ideology, picks up on this latter point and addresses health and disease from a broader perspective. The emphasis here is on taking a long-term perspective on health and disease, and examining disease within societies and different environments, focusing on how these affect our health. The social ideology moves from considering individuals to considering groups of individuals, communities and larger social units, and in doing so, shifts responsibility for health from the individual to social, economic, and political realms. With respect to cancer and prevention of this disease, Robert Proctor (1995) suggests that, 'the value of the social perspective ... is that it allows us to broaden our understanding of where one might intervene in the process of carcinogenesis' (p. 260). Obviously, if the personal responsibility ideology is shaping how we, as individuals and as a society, think of carcinogenesis, we will be focused on individual persons, what predisposes them to get cancer (for example, the breast cancer genes), and what each of these individuals can do to prevent their getting cancer. In contrast, if the social ideology is shaping how we think of carcinogenesis, the focus will necessarily expand from individuals to looking at groups of individuals in conjunction with the environments in which they live and work. New options for preventing cancer, and specifically breast cancer, will present themselves. These options may include creating safer, healthier workplaces and enforcing stricter controls on the disposal of hazardous waste (see Sherwin and Simpson 1999).

Each ideology thus suggests a different approach to the three identified aspects of risk assessment and operates in different ways at the levels of individual persons, scientific research and society. There are dangers in allowing one of these ideologies to dominate the risk discourse and assessment as then only certain features of risk will be attended to and a limited number of options will be available for reducing risk. This emphasizes the necessity of applying a pluralistic ideological approach to risk, so that a variety of risk assessments may be undertaken and a wider number of options for the prevention of breast cancer will be available for both individual women and society. But these general comments about the role of ideology in risk assessment will only start to take hold and become concrete when the specifics of a given controversy about risk and breast cancer prevention are examined. Let us now see how these ideas about the role of ideology(ies) and attention to the different ways risk can be assessed apply in the case of chemoprevention measures.

Practical Application – The Chemoprevention of Breast Cancer

Roughly speaking, chemoprevention is the umbrella term used to describe pharmacological approaches to the prevention of, or the reduction of risk for, a given disease, tamoxifen being by far the most well-known drug used for the prevention of breast cancer. I want now to discuss risk assessment and general risk discourse about tamoxifen and other chemoprevention/hormonal manipulation projects, as well as one possible alternative research route based on the presumed role of oestrogen in the development of breast cancer, in the context of the three previously described ideological perspectives.

Tamoxifen

Tamoxifen (produced by Zeneca Pharmaceuticals under the trade-name Nolvadex) is a drug that was developed initially for the treatment of advanced breast cancer, mainly in those women whose tumours are oestrogen-dependent, and which was also shown to be successful as an adjuvant therapy (Nazari 1994). The chemical structure of tamoxifen is similar to that of oestrogen. It can therefore mimic this hormone and block its binding to tumour cells in the breast, thereby, it is believed, decreasing a tumour's rate of growth or interfering with its replication. Additionally, while tamoxifen is antioestrogenic in the breast, it acts like oestrogen in the rest of the body and therefore may have positive effects on reducing the risks of bone fractures and/or heart disease. Due to tamoxifen's success in treating women with breast cancer, its seeming preventative effect on reducing the recurrence of a patient's original tumour, and its possible prevention of the development of new cancers in the opposite breast of breast cancer patients, the Breast Cancer Prevention Trial (BCPT) was initiated in April 1992 to see whether this drug could be used to prevent breast cancer in healthy women who are at high risk of developing this disease.

There were two groups of women eligible to participate in this clinical trial: one, women over the age of 60 who by age alone were at high risk for breast cancer and, two, women aged 35–59 who were estimated to have a risk of developing breast cancer within the next five years that was equal to or greater than the average risk of a 60-year-old woman. The risk for the younger women was determined by a calculation based on the following factors: the number of first-degree relatives (mother, daughters or sisters) who have been diagnosed as having breast cancer; whether the woman has any children and her age at first delivery; the number of times the woman has had breast lumps biopsied, especially if the tissue was shown to have a condition known as atypical hyperplasia; and the woman's age at her first menstrual period; or a previous diagnosis of the non-invasive breast cancer called lobular carcinoma 'in situ', a disease that greatly increases a woman's chance of developing invasive breast cancer. Participation in the BCPT meant taking either tamoxifen or a placebo twice a day for a period of five years.

This trial was recently ended approximately 14 months early (National Cancer Institute 1998a; Klausner 1998), as the initial study results indicated that high risk women taking tamoxifen showed a 45 per cent reduction in breast cancer incidence as compared to the placebo group. This reduction in breast cancer incidence was relatively constant over the different age groups under study. Taking tamoxifen was also shown to increase the risks, primarily for women over the age of 50, of three rare but life-threatening health problems – endometrial cancer, pulmonary embolism and deep vein thrombosis. An independent Endpoint Review, Safety Monitoring and Advisory Committee concluded that the information on the decreased incidence of breast cancer plus data on the adverse effects of tamoxifen should be released to the BCPT participants. While the results about the decreased incidence of breast cancer are very exciting and suggest that women at high risk have a new option for preventing breast cancer, the conclusion in the National Cancer Institute press release was that, given the risks of taking this drug, the decision to take tamoxifen will need to be a personal/individual one. In other words, taking tamoxifen as a preventative measure may not be appropriate for every woman at high risk:

> As with any medical procedure or intervention, the decision to take tamoxifen is an individual one in which the benefits and risks must be considered ... The choice will vary depending on a woman's age, personal history, family history, and *how she weighs the benefits and risks* (emphasis added). (National Cancer Institute 1998a)

But, given that women can only obtain tamoxifen by prescription, attention must also be directed towards the role physicians will and should play in this decision-making. As will be discussed shortly, uncertainty about how to evaluate these results about tamoxifen also exists at the medical level – thus adding more complexity to this issue.

The final analysis of the BCPT data will be published in scientific journals. But it should be noted that the results of the BCPT, irrespective of the final analysis, cannot be extended to the general population. The results only apply to women who fit the studied risk profiles. Further, the results of this trial probably apply solely to white women with these risk profiles as only approximately 3 per cent of the trial participants were African-American, Asian-American, Hispanic or from other minority ethnic groups (National Cancer Institute 1998a). It is thus extremely difficult to assess what effect tamoxifen may have for women of different ethnicities.

While this news about tamoxifen is encouraging, there are some legitimate concerns to be raised about the risks of this drug as well as its promotion in the media. It is significant that the decision was made to end the trial early and to release the preliminary data to the press and public before the data was peer-reviewed and published.[3] Much of the publicity about tamoxifen has been highly positive – 'this is the new drug for prevention', 'it paves the way for future related drugs', 'the decreased incidence fits with hypotheses about the role of estrogen and estrogen receptors' (National Cancer Institute 1998a) – and even the greater incidence of the three other health problems is couched within comments that increased surveillance for and awareness of these potential problems will help to alleviate or reduce their occurrence and their associated negative outcomes. Finally, the other more common side-effects of tamoxifen experienced by approximately 15–20 per cent of women such as hot flushes, amenorrhoea (irregular menstrual periods), menorrhagia (very heavy menstrual periods), nausea, vomiting, light-headedness and dizziness are rarely mentioned (Goel 1998).

Given this publicity, it is likely that a number of women are asking their physicians about taking this drug. But without published, peer-reviewed results with the full data on the BCPT, how are doctors to advise women and how are women themselves to decide about taking tamoxifen? At both the scientific/medical and individual levels, there is much ambiguity in terms of evaluating the risks and benefits of this drug. Two editorials in the *Canadian Medical Association Journal* help to capture this uncertainty, at the medical level, and offer different possible risk evaluations of the BCPT results. Margolese's (1998) article leans towards optimism with respect to tamoxifen, and urges the reader, the physician, to consider this as one drug with risks among the many other drugs with risks that are taken (focusing on the level of individual decision-making about taking tamoxifen). Goel's article (1998) is more reserved in its praise for tamoxifen and suggests that the use of tamoxifen outside of clinical trials should be discouraged until more is known about its risks and benefits (focusing more on the level of the scientific research agenda). The role of ideology in shaping judgements about tamoxifen's risks and benefits is dramatically emphasized by these two articles: Margolese implicitly endorses the technology ideology by attending more to the positive outcomes of the BCPT, namely the reduced incidence of breast cancer. He also points to the benefits of the continuing trials and research on drugs related to tamoxifen and other possible chemoprevention agents, such as growth factors and retinoid, and concludes by comparing taking tamoxifen with the risks of taking the birth control pill and hormonal replacement therapy, two drugs which a number of women use, and suggesting that tamoxifen is not all that different from these latter drugs in terms of the risks each drug poses. In contrast, Goel's paper has a more cautious tone; in part, I believe, because he wants to use a broader perspective for evaluating tamoxifen (perhaps being somewhat sceptical of the technology ideology). Much of Goel's paper is an attempt to find tamoxifen's place within the various possible approaches to breast cancer prevention, such as changing lifestyle patterns or prophylactic mastectomy. Goel points to the need for developing guidelines for tamoxifen's use; he notes that these guidelines will require input from both public health agencies and breast cancer treatment groups. Finally, he emphasizes the importance of generating decision support tools for consumers, i.e. individual women interested in taking tamoxifen, and physicians based on these guidelines, thereby demonstrating one of the ways in which communication between the social, scientific and individual levels of risk discourse can take place.

But, as if things were not already hard enough to sort out, the results of two other trials on tamoxifen were recently published in *The Lancet,* which contradict those of the BCPT and claim that tamoxifen had no demonstrable effect on the incidence of breast cancer (Veronesi 1998; Powles 1998). The publication of these results has spurred speculation about why contradictions between the data from these three studies exist: are the groups of women studied sufficiently different, that is, do they have different risks for developing breast cancer such that one would not expect the same results from taking tamoxifen? In a commentary published with the results of the British and Italian trials on tamoxifen, Kathleen Pritchard (1998: 81) suggests that,

> [t]he seemingly different results reported today may be largely due to a younger population in both [the British and Italian] trials ... to differences in the populations studied (most importantly, those in risk levels and in family history).

She concludes that the rush, at least in some places, to prescribe tamoxifen is premature and advocates the continuing study of tamoxifen, again focusing on what the future research agenda should be (the International Breast Cancer Intervention study is currently underway on tamoxifen). Finally, as Pritchard and others have suggested, although the results of the BCPT may be encouraging in terms of the possible decreased incidence of breast cancer, the real endpoint for these studies should be the effects, if any, of taking tamoxifen on mortality. It may be that taking tamoxifen only delays the onset of breast cancer rather than truly preventing it – continued follow-up on women taking tamoxifen is required in order to answer these types of questions.

As the above discussion indicates, depending on which level of the risk discourse is applied, and which ideological approach is dominant, different evaluations of the preventative potential of tamoxifen can be arrived at. At the scientific level, there is agreement on the need for continuing research on tamoxifen given the ambiguous results, yet there is also disagreement with respect to the weight that should be attached to these disparate results. There is seemingly little consensus at both the scientific/medical and social levels as to whether tamoxifen should be prescribed or recommended for high-risk women; in fact, the decision-making role about tamoxifen has primarily been placed on individual women. In light of the uncertainty about tamoxifen's ability to prevent breast cancer though, it seems reasonable to ask if this is a fair choice to ask women to make – should personal responsibility for avoiding breast cancer extend to taking this newest drug? Medicine is offering what it deems to be the best available measure for preventing breast cancer, at least until new drugs without these side-effects are found; each woman is asked to decide whether she agrees that tamoxifen is a suitable answer for her.

A further complication in relation to the risk assessment of tamoxifen use at both the personal and scientific/medical levels relates to the uncertainties involved in determining any individual woman's risk of developing breast cancer. It is extremely difficult accurately to translate population statistics to individual statistics; in addition, the identified risk factors for breast cancer only account for approximately 30 per cent of all breast cancer cases and, as a result, even if a woman has one or more of these risk factors, it is never really clear that these actually are what caused or contributed to her getting breast cancer (Henderson 1993). In an article on assessing individual risk for breast cancer, Anne McTiernan, Mary Ann Gilligan and Carol Redmond (1997: 647) conclude that 'risk assessment [for developing an individual woman's risk profile], while a promising tool for research now, and for clinical areas in the future, is still too imprecise for accurate prediction of breast cancer occurrence in individuals'. Thus, even though all women are technically at some level of risk for developing breast cancer, the authors suggest that trying to put a specific number on this risk is difficult as well as possibly dangerous (in that an estimate that is too high may unnecessarily cause great anxiety while an underestimate may falsely reassure). Thus, an additional layer of uncertainty is added to the risk evaluation of tamoxifen.

Expanding the Focus?

The broader implications of this focus on 'the new drug' for the prevention of breast cancer also need to be considered. One concern about the hype surrounding tamoxifen deals with the type of prevention being promoted by this highly publicized research: prevention based on drug-taking by (currently) healthy women. This approach to

breast cancer prevention is based on a risk evaluation at the population level which suggests that the risks posed by this pharmacological
intervention are counterbalanced by the high risk for some women of
developing breast cancer. While it is true that chemoprevention
measures may help prevent some women from getting breast cancer,
this reliance on drugs to prevent disease does increase the dependence
of women on medicine and helps to reinforce the technology ideology. As Richard Klausner, the Director of the National Cancer
Institute, stated in his report to the Senate Appropriations
Subcommittee on Labour, Health, Human Services, and Related
Agencies about the outcome of the BCPT:

> This emphasis on individual risk is important. Our ability to iden-
> tify individuals at risk for disease and to begin to rationally
> intervene, based upon our knowledge of the disease process, is
> what medicine will become. (Klausner 1998)

In turn Dr Adrian Fugh-Berman (1994: 111) comments that, 'the
Tamoxifen and Proscar [a potential preventative drug being tested for
prostrate cancer] trials point to an alarming fact: Doctors are now
suggesting that simply being a man or woman puts one at sufficient
risk for pharmaceutical intervention'. Is this the kind of society we
want to live in? The social implications of this emphasis on the technology ideology in conjunction with the personal responsibility
ideology raise several important questions.

This intense focus on individuals in terms of risk and prevention of
disease is further evidenced by what has been described as 'the
medicalization of risk.'

> until the different dimensions of risk are fully recognized and made
> legitimate [such as social and environmental influences], clinical
> control over the uncertainty [about risk] through the medicaliza-
> tion of risk will only increase. (Gifford 1986: 240)

> patients undergo medical procedures that are potentially dangerous
> or unnecessary, even though none of the patients is sick. Marc
> Micozzi, M.D., Ph.D., director of the National Museum of Health
> and Medicine and an authority on diet and cancer, calls it 'the
> medicalization of prevention'. With this approach, doctors tell
> their patients, 'Detecting – and treating – diseases at their earliest
> stages may save your life'. (Fugh-Berman 1994: 84)

Whether it is termed medicalization of risk or of prevention, the ideological commitments are the same. These commitments are: (a) to the new technologies that allow us to discover information about the aetiology and development of disease and that allow us to intervene at earlier and earlier stages of disease – now even before a disease occurs, that is, when one is at risk of getting a disease; and (b) to the individual's responsibility to take advantage of these opportunities for preventing disease. The presence of these new technologies and pharmacologies suggests that, since science has developed the means of intervening and potentially altering a person's risk profile, we, as individuals, should (and must?) take advantage of these opportunities. The underlying assumption is that the earlier one can intervene in the disease process (even before it starts), the greater one's chances will be of avoiding something 'bad' in the future, the something bad in this case being breast cancer. While in general this assumption is probably true, it does not mean that the early interventions undertaken do not carry their own set of risks. Recall the risks of taking tamoxifen; how does one balance the risks of taking this drug *now* against the risk of developing breast cancer *later*? Margaret Lock (1996: 12) suggests that these interventions and constant attention on one's risk profile lead to 'a culturally enhanced anxiety, one peculiarly evident in North America, which encourages middle class women, at least, to see the body as inherently valuable and ever in need of protection and modification through technological intervention'. Additional sources of this anxiety could include regarding women who get breast cancer as failures – failures for not having caught it sooner or changed their lifestyle accordingly – and the myth that medicine can 'cure all' or even 'prevent all' with its drugs and technological interventions. These attitudes ensure that the focus is on each individual woman's responsibility to do everything possible to avoid getting breast cancer, but 'everything' in this case refers to a (continued) reliance on the medical establishment.

The main problem with this focus on the pharmacological manipulation of risk is that it results in a situation that can restrict, rather than open up, the options for women to reduce their risk of developing breast cancer. Although more information is needed to help resolve the current ambiguity about the benefits and risks of tamoxifen, there is a danger that an increasing portion of the research agenda may be devoted to this drug and others like it, making it very difficult for alternative forms of prevention or risk questions to be investigated. It is worth, again, asking whose interests and values are being served by and are determining these research routes. Are women who have and could potentially get breast cancer at the forefront of this decision-making or do profit motives have a strong(er) influence? Indeed, tamoxifen and related future drugs are not the only chemo-prevention routes being investigated for reducing the risk of breast cancer. Given the presumed role of oestrogen in stimulating the promotion of a transformed cell into an active breast cancer, research has been directed towards other interventions for altering women's exposure to oestrogen. One such project has been proposed by researchers in California; this hormonal manipulation project

> suppresses ovarian function and replaces ovarian hormones with a synthetic hormonal formula [reducing ovulation to approximately three times per year]. The regimen is being tested as a contraceptive that might collaterally reduce breast cancer risk. (Waller and Batt 1995: 830; see also Spicer and Pike 1994)

Other possible suggestions for chemoprevention include inducing false pregnancies by hormonal measures in teenagers/young women to allow them to benefit from the protective effects of pregnancy while not actually having a child (Rennie 1993: 42).

These potential chemoprevention measures involve a greater degree of hormonal manipulation of women's bodies and have therefore attracted particular attention and opposition from breast cancer advocacy groups. While breast cancer advocacy groups do not dispute the fact that these projects may be a potential way of reducing the risk of getting breast cancer, there is a principled objection to this research focus, due both to the increased medical intervention and thus medicalized control it requires, as well as recognition of the other health risks these measures pose (see Rennie 1993; Fugh-Berman 1994). Although evidence does point to the fact that a woman's breasts are more susceptible to damage or to the effects of oestrogen and carcinogens during development and/or before pregnancy, should this entail young women being exposed to these drastic forms of hormonal manipulation? Do we want to support the technology ideology to this extent? Especially when the understanding of breast cancer and the female body is incomplete, advocacy groups argue that these forms of hormonal manipulation seem to jump to the high-tech pharmacological solution much too quickly. If one needs to 'alter' the individual, advocacy groups indicate that they would prefer focusing on diet, exercise and other lifestyle factors, before turning to these forms of manipulation. The risks of these forms of prevention are very low and their benefits carry over into many other areas of health. In addition, advocacy groups emphasize the need to get away from solely considering the individual's responsibility for health. They want to expand the focus to include changes that could be made to the environment and in our societies and point to the need for collective responsibility and change. These groups force us to ask, at all levels of risk discourse, whether the risks of breast cancer are sufficient to warrant manipulation of very young women's hormonal systems and whether we, as individuals and as a society, necessarily want an increasing array of medications for 'reducing' risk. In interrogating research priorities, who sets them and what is motivating these decisions, breast cancer advocacy groups help to bring the social ideology to the forefront as a counter-balance to the technology ideology and to shift the focus of the personal responsibility ideology. This revised focus of the personal ideology emphasizes the role of individual women in promoting the social ideology, that is, to put pressure on the social and scientific levels of risk discourse and assessment to consider options other than those currently pursued under the technology ideology. Breast cancer advocacy groups point out that this new perspective does not believe that all technology is bad, but that rather than always developing technologies with an eye to changing the individual (whether it is by drugs or new surgeries), technology should be used to improve the environment and our societies.

A Different Strategy for Breast Cancer Prevention

If the social ideology is used to provide the context for breast cancer risk assessment, a different way of thinking about risk and the various approaches that can be taken to reducing the occurrence of this disease begins to become more apparent. For example, given the post-industrial society in which we live replete with its manufactured chemicals, it is more than likely that these chemicals contribute to the risk(s) of developing breast cancer and other diseases. There are many chemicals in today's world that mimic oestrogen and have been shown to have an effect on the reproductive system and, as a result, may be playing a role in breast cancer incidence. Indeed, there is adequate preliminary evidence for supporting a thesis that the causes of breast cancer are more diverse than the current approach, with its emphasis on individual causation, suggests, and that breast cancer advocacy groups are right in trying to encourage this wider socio-environmental approach to breast cancer. A paper by Devra Lee Davis and H. Leon Bradlow (1995) titled 'Can Environmental Estrogens Cause Breast Cancer?' concluded that, while xenoestrogens (foreign oestrogens) cannot account for all cases of breast cancer, they do represent a preventable cause. These authors gave an overview of their research in this area as well as including evidence from many other studies about xenoestrogens. A list of chemicals known as xenoestrogens includes: chlorinated organic compounds (e.g. DDT, atrazine), plastics (bisphenol A), pharmaceuticals (synthetic oestrogens – HRT, oral contraceptives) and fuel constituents (aromatic hydrocarbons). Research has shown that these chemicals do have oestrogenic properties in the body, and emphasizes that there are many more external sources of oestrogen beyond HRT and oral contraceptives about which we should be concerned. Currently, research is being conducted to discover whether the other listed chemicals can be implicated in the cause of breast cancer; so far, DDT and some PCBs seem to have a role. Since many of these compounds persist for a long time in the environment (for example, DDT persists for approximately 50 years), this magnifies the need for action now on the hypothesis that these chemicals may be a cause of breast cancer as well as other health problems such as infertility. It is also very likely that other, non-oestrogenic, chemicals can contribute to breast cancer occurrence. The connection between carcinogens and breast cancer may be unclear, but not unlikely. When one considers the fact that it is known that the breasts are susceptible to external factors during development, concern about exposure to carcinogenic and oestrogenic chemicals seems justified (see also Hall 1995; Montague 1995).

Viewed from this broader socio-environmental perspective, it becomes apparent that tamoxifen and other forms of chemoprevention are, in a sense, basically only stop-gap measures or temporary solutions, in that they can only help individual women in the short term. The taking of drugs or other such options, without making any long-term socio-environmental changes, will need to be repeated for each generation of women and this seems to miss the alternative environmental approach that can concurrently be taken to reducing breast cancer risk. Chemoprevention measures cannot fully address the long-term perspective that is also needed for dealing with breast cancer risk and for making changes that will help to reduce everyone's risk of disease in the future.[4] Ruth Hubbard agrees with the broader approach to disease and health suggested by the social ideology:

our state of health depends not only on what goes on inside our bodies, but also on the conditions under which we live and work. Individual susceptibilities may play a part, but many of the preconditions for our health are beyond the control of any but a privileged few ...

[Many] seem to think 'prevention' involves mainly the behavioral choices that relatively affluent individuals are in a position to make, rather than the economic, public health, and medical measures that would reduce unnecessary risks and improve everyone's chance to be healthy. An excessive preoccupation with individual concerns and responsibilities is detrimental to health when it encourages us, as a society, to neglect the systemic conditions that affect all of us. (Hubbard 1997: 61, 63)

Conclusion

Thus it is apparent that the identification of different ideological perspectives has a vital role in risk assessment and risk discourse. If one ideology dominates the process of risk assessment, only certain questions about risk will be asked and only a limited number of options for reducing that risk will be developed. By applying the conceptual framework developed in the first section of this chapter to chemoprevention measures for breast cancer, it is apparent that attending to the influence of ideologies in risk discourse and risk assessment is vital both to understanding different evaluations of risk (for example, as with the benefits and harms of tamoxifen) and ensuring that alternative approaches to prevention are given their due consideration. The discussion here suggests that we, as participants in the different levels of risk discourse and risk assessment, have an obligation to acknowledge and be aware of how ideologies shape our own understanding of risk and influence the approaches to breast cancer prevention that are taken. Further, it seems imperative that effort also be made at each level of risk discourse to include a plurality of ideological perspectives – particularly at the scientific and social levels as a narrowing of perspectives at these levels will necessarily limit the options available for individual women to prevent breast cancer. Finally, given that the technology and personal responsibility ideologies tend to have more currency in risk discourse and that, as a result, the approaches suggested by these ideologies for the prevention of breast cancer may be the ones typically expected or more readily accepted, it becomes clear that the long-term changes suggested by the social ideology will be difficult to implement. But, a balancing out or a redirection in the current strategies for breast cancer prevention seems to be necessary if a continued and increasing dependence on the medical establishment is to be avoided. New drugs and new technologies may be helpful, but in addition to these forms of prevention, the environments in which we all live, work, and play need to be cleaned-up; not only to help prevent breast cancer, but other diseases as well.

Notes

1   Many thanks are extended to Dr Susan Sherwin, Department of Philosophy, Dalhousie University for her helpful suggestions and input on this chapter. And, although the following discussion is written primarily from a North American perspective, it is my hope that the ideas and arguments contained within will serve to both challenge and inform women from a broad range of cultural and social backgrounds.
2   Individuals can also organize themselves into interest groups based on, for example, a common social or political goal. By doing so, this may create a fourth level of risk discourse. However, this added layer of discourse will not be addressed separately in this chapter.
3   One thing that should not be ignored is the very real profit that can be made from successfully marketing this drug. It is estimated that approximately 29 million women in the United States alone fall into the 'high-risk' category and could conceivably take this drug (see National Cancer Institute 1998b).
4   This is not to say that chemoprevention measures should be abandoned altogether though, for until and even when environments are cleaned up and made safe, these options will need to be available.

References

Brunk, C., L. Haworth, and B. Lee. 'Is a Scientific Assessment of Risk Possible? Value Assumptions in the Canadian Alachor Controversy'. *Dialogue* XXX (1991) pp. 235–47.
Cranor, C. F. 'Some Moral Issues in Risk Assessment' *Ethics* 101 (October 1990) pp. 123–43.
Davis, D.L., and H. L. Bradlow. 'Can Environmental Estrogens Cause Breast Cancer?' *Scientific American* (October 1995) pp. 166–71.
Fugh-Berman, A. 'The New Dangers of Medical Prevention'. *Natural Health* (March/April 1994) pp. 84–5, 111–12.
Gifford, S., C. Janes and R. Stall. *Anthropology and Epidemiology – Interdisciplinary Approaches to the Study of Health and Risk* (Boston: D. Reidel Publishing Company 1986).

Goel, V. 'Tamoxifen and Breast Cancer Prevention: What Should You Tell Your Patients?' *Canadian Medical Association Journal* 158(12) (16 June 1998) pp. 1615–17.

Hansson, S. O. 1993. 'The False Promises of Risk Analysis'. *Ratio* (New Series) VI (1 June 1993) pp. 16–26.

Hall, R. H. 'Female Biology, Toxic Chemicals, and Preventing Breast Cancer: A Path Not Taken'. Presented at *The International Conference on Breast Cancer and the Environment* (3–4 November 1995): Niagara Falls, Ontario, Canada.

Henderson, I. C. 'Risk Factors for Breast Cancer Development'. *American Cancer Society* (15 March 1993). United States: Professional Education Publication.

Hubbard, R., and E. Wald. *Exploding the Gene Myth* (Boston: Beacon Press 1997).

Klausner M.D., and R.D. Klausner 'Breast Cancer Prevention Trial', Given before the Senate Appropriations Subcommittee on Labor, Health, Human Services, and Related Agencies. (21 April 1998). http:www.nci.nih.gov/legis/trials/html

Lock, M. 'Social and Cultural Issues in Connection with Breast Cancer Testing and Screening'. Paper prepared for *International Association of Bioethics* conference (on file with author). Montreal: McGill University (1996)

Margolese, R. 'How Do We Interpret the Results of the Breast Cancer Prevention Trial?', *Canadian Medical Association Journal* 158(12) (16 June 1998) pp. 1613–14.

Martin, R. M. *The Philosopher's Dictionary* (second edition) (Ontario, Canada: Broadview Press 1994).

McTiernan, A., M.A. Gilligan and C. Redmond. 'Assessing Individual Risk for Breast Cancer: Risky Business'. *Journal of Clinical Epidemiology* 50(5) (1997) pp. 647–56.

Montague, P. 'Making Good Decisions'. *Rachel's Environment and Health Weekly* (30 November 1995). Annapolis, Maryland, United States: Environmental Research Foundation.

National Cancer Institute. 'Breast Cancer Prevention Trial Shows Major Benefit, Some Risk'. *Press Release* (Monday, 6 April 1998a). http://rex.nci.nih.gov/massmedia/pressreleases/ prevtrial.htm.

National Cancer Institute. 'Charts and Graphs – BCPT Conclusions' (1998b). http://rex.nci.hih.gov/massmedia/pressreleases/prevtrial GRAPHS2.htm#anchor163691471.

Nazari M.D., Nancy E. *Letter from Zeneca Pharmaceuticals Concerning Tamoxifen.* (Wilmington, United States: Zeneca Pharmaceuticals Group 1994).

Powles, T., R. Eeles, S. Ashley et al., 'Interim Analysis of the Incidence of Breast Cancer in the Royal Marsden Hospital Tamoxifen Randomized Chemoprevention Trial'. *The Lancet* 352(9122) (1998) pp. 98–101.

Pritchard, K. 'Commentary: Is Tamoxifen Effective in Prevention of Breast Cancer'. *The Lancet* 352(9122) (1998) pp. 80–1.

Proctor, R. N. *Cancer Wars: How Politics Shape What We Know and Don't Know About Cancer* (New York: Basic Books 1995).

Rennie, S. 'Breast Cancer Prevention: Diet vs. Drugs', *Ms.* 38 (May/June 1993) pp. 38–46.

Sherwin, S., and C. Simpson. 'Ethical Questions in the Pursuit of Genetic Information: Geneticization and BRCA1'. In A. Thompson and R. Chadwick, eds. *Genetic Information: Acquisition, Access and Control* (London: Plenum

Publishing Company 1999).

Shrader-Frechette, K.S. *Risk and Rationality* (Berkeley: University of California Press 1991).

Spicer, D.V. and M.C. Pike. 'Sex Steroids and Breast Cancer Prevention'. *Monograph National Cancer Institute* 16 (1994) pp. 139–47.

Veronesi, P., P. Maisonneuve, A. Costa et al. 'Prevention of Breast Cancer with Tamoxifen: Preliminary Findings from the Italian Randomized Trial among Hysterectomized Women'. *The Lancet* 352(9122) (1998) pp. 93–7.

Waller, M. and S. Batt. 'Advocacy Groups for Breast Cancer Patients'. *Canadian Medical Association Journal* 152(6) (1995) pp. 829–33.

Webster's Ninth New Collegiate Dictionary. (Ontario, Canada: Thomas Allen & Son Ltd 1989).

6
Reconstructing the Body or Reconstructing the Woman? Perceptions of Prophylactic Mastectomy for Hereditary Breast Cancer Risk

Nina Hallowell

During the last decade of the twentieth century we have witnessed an ever-increasing 'geneticisation' of life (Lippman 1992). In addition to certain common diseases, such as cancer, diabetes and heart disease, more and more aspects of life are said to be influenced by our genetic endowment, for example, maternal behaviour, homosexuality and alcoholism. The geneticization and the concomitant 'medicalization' (Zola 1972; Illich 1975) of behaviour and disease have profound social, political and ethical ramifications, for both individuals and society (The Nuffield Council on Bioethics 1993, 1998). This chapter focuses on some of the implications of the geneticization of a common disease – breast cancer. It explores what it means for women to be identified, and to identify themselves, as 'at risk' of hereditary breast cancer (HBC).

Of the 30,000 cases of breast cancer which are diagnosed in the United Kingdom each year, between 5 and 10 per cent are thought to be caused by an inherited predisposition. Some of the genetic mutations responsible for causing this type of cancer have recently been identified (BRCA1, Miki et al. 1994; BRCA2, Wooster et al. 1994). It is calculated that carriers of BRCA2 mutations have a 75 per cent lifetime risk of developing breast cancer (Tonin et al. 1995) while BRCA1 mutation carriers have an 85 per cent lifetime risk of breast cancer and an ovarian cancer risk which may be as high as 60 per cent (Easton et al. 1995). Women who have a family history of breast cancer are referred for genetic counselling, where their risks of inheriting a genetic mutation and developing this disease are calculated and different types of risk management are discussed.

At present the identification of a woman's genetic risk status is usually based on the type of family history she presents (i.e. the number, type and ages of affected relatives in her family). Although predictive DNA testing for an inherited predisposition to breast cancer is now available, testing is not widespread. Technically this is a difficult procedure, and these tests are normally confined to women from multi-case families once the mutation has been identified in their affected relatives.

Although only a very few women receive genetic confirmation of their risk status many more women are identified as being 'at risk' of hereditary breast cancer because of their family history. All at risk women, i.e. confirmed and potential carriers of the mutated gene, are encouraged to adopt breast cancer risk management practices. One option offered to (potential) mutation carriers is annual breast screening, i.e. mammography (or breast ultrasound) plus clinical breast examination. The rationale for screening high-risk women is that cancers may be identified at an early stage when the prognosis is good, thus reducing the risk of dying from cancer. However, at the present time there are no data to indicate that breast screening is effective in reducing mortality in high-risk groups (Neugut and Jacobson 1995). Indeed, breast screening itself carries 'risks' for high-risk women, and offers no guarantee of protection from the disease. First, cancers may occur during the interval between appointments. Second, screening may not detect cancers, indeed, it is widely accepted that mammography is less effective in detecting cancers in younger women because of the density of the breast tissue. Third, screening may have iatrogenic consequences. As Jofesson (1998) notes, the rate of false positives (in low-risk populations) is significant, and this may result in women having unnecessary exploratory operations. Furthermore, it has been calculated that annual exposure to radiation may compound the risk of developing breast cancer in gene carriers (Den Otter et al. 1996).

Alternatively, at-risk women can take steps to decrease their risk by undergoing prophylactic surgery – bilateral mastectomy. Recent evidence suggests that prophylactic mastectomy confers a significant reduction in breast cancer risk (Hartmann et al. 1997). However, as it is impossible to guarantee the removal of all the breast tissue, even in those cases were breast reconstruction is not planned, there is a residual risk of developing cancer following surgery. Indeed, breast cancers have been documented as occurring following prophylactic mastectomy (Ziegler and Kroll 1991). Furthermore, there are medical risks associated with this procedure, such as the risks associated with anaesthesia, post-operative complications such as infections and, in the case of women who opt for breast reconstruction, there is ongoing debate about the risks of connective tissue disease associated with silicon breast implants (Cooper and Dennison 1998).

Finally, it must be noted that, in addition to the physical costs, these forms of risk management may also carry psychological costs. Several studies have explored the emotional well-being of high-risk women attending screening programmes for breast cancer. These suggest that screening may increase anxiety (Kash et al. 1992; Lerman and Schwartz 1993). The psychosocial effects of undergoing prophy-lactic surgery are less well documented, although there is evidence to suggest that women who undergo prophylactic surgery do experience a decrease in cancer worries (Stephanek et al. 1995). One of the prob-lems with these studies is that little is known of the long-term psychological consequences of this type of surgery.

Thus, despite the fact that only a small proportion of women are thought to carry genetic mutations which predispose them to develop cancer, the geneticization of breast cancer has led to the recategoriza-tion of many healthy women (and their offspring) as 'at risk' – 'potentially sick, potentially vulnerable and potentially stigmatized' (Kenen 1994: 49). However, as the above discussion suggests, it is not only an individual's health status that may be affected by the geneti-cization of this disease, but also their health and psychological well-being, for the geneticization of breast cancer has meant that many healthy women have been encouraged to adopt risk manage-ment practices which may have iatrogenic consequences. In this chapter I will look at how a group of women who have been identified as 'at risk' perceive their genetic risks and a particular form of risk management – bilateral prophylactic mastectomy. I will argue that the adoption of an 'at risk' identity has profound implications for the way these women conceive of the self and their bodies, which in turn influences their decisions about risk management. However, before proceeding any further, I think it is appropriate to outline the theo-retical background which informs the subsequent analysis.

Genetic knowledge = dangerous knowledge?

Genetic risks constitute 'corporeal' or 'embodied' risks (Kavanagh and Broom 1998). Corporeal risks are distinguished from environmental risks, such as atmospheric pollution, and lifestyle risks, such as smoking, on the basis that they are internalized, they derive from, and are located within, individuals' bodies. According to Kavanagh and Broom (1998), because corporeal risks originate in the body they may be perceived as less avoidable than lifestyle or environmental risks, and this is potentially threatening to the self. Using data collected during a study of women identified as at risk of cervical cancer as a result of an abnormal pap smear, they observe that the experience of living with corporeal risk is characterized by a Cartesian splitting of body and self in which corporeal risk is experienced as of the body but not of the self. Kavanagh and Broom argue that the construction of the body as 'other' is perceived as necessary for living with one's risk status, for without this objectification of the body the self would also be experienced as at risk. Furthermore, they note that this disconnection of body and self facilitates the management of corporeal risk, in so far as it means that risk management – the surveillance, or disposal, of at-risk body parts – is not perceived as having any implications for the self.

Kavanagh and Broom acknowledge that the disconnection between body and self they observed has not been reported in studies of other types of embodied risk (for example, hypertension and high serum cholesterol). This observation has led them to speculate that the process they describe is intrinsically related to the type of risk involved in their study, namely cancer risk. They observe that in Western societies cancer is commonly constructed as 'other' and frequently portrayed as an 'invader' of bodies (see, for example, Sontag 1979; Stacey, 1997), and argue that these cultural constructions of cancer may in some way be responsible for the Cartesian splitting observed in their participants' accounts. However, this explanation is contradicted by evidence from empirical studies of women who have undergone therapeutic mastectomy for breast cancer. This research suggests that although some women do talk about a fragmentation of self and body during treatment for breast cancer, they also experience the loss of a body part – in this case a cancerous breast – as having a profound effect on the self, and report that mastectomy necessitates a reconstruction of self-identity (Langelleir and Sullivan 1998).

Although it is possible that the experience of being at risk of cancer is not the same as having a cancer, it is also possible that it is not the type of risk that is responsible for the disconnection Kavanagh and Broom describe, but the location of risk within the body i.e, reproductive organs, in this case, the cervix. Indeed, Martin (1989) reports a similar disassociation between body and self in her analysis of women's accounts of menstruation, childbirth and menopause. She observes that the social construction of the reproductive body in biomedical discourses is recapitulated in women's accounts of their reproductive experiences. Thus, the reproductive body is objectified, it is perceived as uncontrollable and therefore separate from the self.

If it is accepted that the body is socially constructed (for example, Martin 1989; Bartky 1990), then it can be argued that different body parts may have a different significance for individuals, in terms of the role they assume in the construction of self-identity. If this is the case, then as the above research suggests, it may be easier for individuals to objectify some body parts, namely internal or invisible parts (for example, the ovaries, uterus and cervix) than others (for example, external or visible parts (breasts)). Bearing this argument in mind, in this chapter I will explore how individuals conceive of and manage another type of corporeal risk – hereditary breast cancer (HBC). Using six case studies of women identified as at risk of HBC, I describe how these women understand their risk of developing cancer and how they regard prophylactic bilateral mastectomy. I will argue that the self and the body are constructed as internally related (i.e. the self is under-stood as necessarily embodied) within their accounts; in so far as the management of breast cancer risk by prophylactic surgery is seen as necessarily having implications for self-identity.

The Studies

This chapter is based on a subset of interviews collected during two qualitative studies of women with a family history of breast and/or ovarian cancer. The first was carried out during 1994–7, and was an evaluation of genetic counselling for hereditary breast/ovarian cancer (HBOC). This included pre- and post clinic interviews and observa-tions of genetic counselling sessions. These interviews concentrated on the following: risk perception, understanding of the cancer family history, experiences of counselling, perceptions of the different risk management options and subsequent risk management decisions.

The second study commenced in 1998 and is ongoing. This research investigates the psychosocial implications of undergoing prophylactic oophorectomy for hereditary ovarian cancer risk. The face-to-face interviews are open-ended but address the following topics: experi-ences of genetic counselling, family history, risk perception, surgical decision-making, and perceptions and implications of prophylactic surgery.

This chapter focuses on six case studies of women who had actively pursued the idea of prophylactic mastectomy following genetic counselling for HBC. Tracey, Mandy, Sarah and Sue had sought further advice either from breast surgeons or genetic counsellors about what prophylactic surgery involved and whether they should pursue this option. Victoria and Patricia had undergone a prophylactic mastectomy plus breast reconstruction because of their genetic risk. Tracey, Mandy, Patricia and Sarah were recruited from the Family History clinic in Cambridge and Sue and Tracey were recruited from the United Kingdom Co-ordinating Committee for Cancer Research's Familial Ovarian Cancer Register. The mean age of the participants was 36 years. None was being treated for breast cancer or had had any form of cancer in the past. Tracey, Sarah, Mandy and Patricia had a family history of breast cancer and Sue and Victoria had a family history of both breast and ovarian cancer. With the exception of Victoria, none of these women had been offered DNA testing.

Tracey (24 years) is a full-time student. She is single and in a long-term heterosexual relationship. She has no children. Her family history of breast cancer includes a sister who died of breast cancer at the age of 26 and her grandmother and two aunts who were affected with breast cancer. During genetic counselling she was given a 20 per cent lifetime risk of developing breast cancer. In the year following genetic counselling she visited a breast surgeon to discuss prophylactic mastectomy. He persuaded her to delay the decision to undergo the operation. During this visit she also had the opportunity to talk to a woman who had undergone a prophylactic mastectomy some years previously, and had set up a support group for women who have had or were considering this operation. She is currently having annual breast screening (ultrasound and clinical breast examination).

Sarah (33 years) runs an import business with her partner. She has been living with him for a few years and was arranging their wedding at the time of the interview. They have no children and are not planning to have any at present. Sarah has a family history of breast cancer; her mother died from breast cancer at the age of 42 and her sister developed breast cancer aged 28 and was in the terminal stages of secondary lung cancer when I interviewed Sarah. During genetic counselling she was given a lifetime risk of developing breast cancer of 33 per cent. She had contacted the genetic counsellor after her appointment to ask further questions about surgery. She said that she was going to discuss this option with a breast surgeon. She was also going to contact Tracey to talk about this option and get a contact address for the support group. She is currently having annual breast screening (ultrasound and clinical breast examination).

Mandy (40 years old) is an academic. She is married with two sons. Her family history of breast cancer included her brother who was diagnosed with breast cancer the age of 54 and was being treated for secondary lung cancer at the time she was interviewed and her mother who had been successfully treated for breast cancer twenty years earlier. Mandy could not recall the risk estimate she was given in the clinic. She had visited a breast surgeon a couple of years previously to discuss mastectomy, but was still undecided about taking this course of action. She is currently having annual breast screening (mammography and clinical breast examination).

Sue (41 years) works as a part-time childminder. She lives with her partner and they have two sons (7 and 5 years). Her family history of ovarian and breast cancer included her mother who died of ovarian cancer at 50 years, a sister who died of ovarian cancer at 49 and two sisters who had breast cancer in their forties, one of whom was undergoing treatment at the time of the interview. Sue had genetic counselling six years ago, but could not remember the risks she had been given. She underwent a prophylactic oophorectomy at 37 years and discussed prophylactic mastectomy with a surgeon last year. She says that he persuaded her that surgery was unnecessary. She is currently undergoing annual breast screening (mammography and clinical breast examination).

Victoria (38 years) runs a business with her partner. She is married and has a daughter (18 years) and two sons (9 and 7 years). Her mother died of ovarian cancer at the age of 50, her sister had breast cancer and died of ovarian cancer at 43. In addition two of her aunts died of ovarian and breast cancer, respectively. Victoria had a BRCA1 predictive test when she was 37 years old and was found to carry a mutation. She was given an 85 per cent risk of developing breast cancer and a 60 per cent risk of ovarian cancer during her lifetime. During the following year she had a prophylactic oophorectomy (plus hysterectomy) and a bilateral prophylactic mastectomy with breast reconstruction (implants plus nipple conservation) two months later.

Patricia (41 years) is in the process of divorcing her husband. She has no children and previously has undergone two cycles of IVF. Her mother developed breast cancer at 45 and died of secondary bone cancer at 57. Other affected relatives included an aunt and grandmother who died of breast cancer, and an uncle who was successfully treated for breast cancer nine years ago. Patricia reported that the genetic counsellor had given her a breast cancer risk of 'upwards of 25 per cent' during her lifetime. She had undergone a bilateral prophylactic mastectomy with breast reconstruction (implants plus nipple conservation) two years before the interview.

A thematic analysis of the interviews was undertaken to establish the meaning of risk and risk management (specifically, prophylactic mastectomy) for these women. The categories were initially guided by the interview topics and emerging themes were then identified and refined. Atlas-ti (Muhr 1994), a qualitative analysis software package, was used to manage the data. The analysis revealed that these women draw on two competing discourses when discussing their attitudes about prophylactic surgery: the *dangerous body* in which the body is constructed as a site of risk, a dangerous object which is more or less amenable to control, and the *feminine body* in which the body is constructed as naturally gendered. I will argue that the tensions generated by these two discourses not only influence their decisions about whether to proceed with prophylactic surgery, but may also influence their adjustment to this procedure.

Genetic Bodies = Dangerous Bodies

The ... point is not that everything is bad, but that everything is dangerous ... If everything is dangerous, then we always have something to do. (Foucault 1984: 343)

During genetic counselling for hereditary breast cancer the body is objectified as a collection of genes, and particular body parts (breasts) are defined as sites of risk. In so far as the main aim of counselling is to determine the probability that an individual carries a 'faulty' or 'mutated' gene, the discourse of the clinic constructs the body as a set of probabilities – the probability that it is defective and the further probability that this defect will result in a life-threatening cancer. Thus, during these clinical encounters, the body is normalized as a risky or defective object, which must be controlled or altered through surveillance (mammographic/ultrasonic screening) or prophylactic surgery (bilateral mastectomy).

In contrast with clinicians, the women who took part in this research did not construct their bodies as risky or defective objects, but as dangerous. The risk of breast cancer was not conceived as a neutral probability, but as an ever-present danger within their lives (Douglas and Wildavsky 1988; Douglas 1992). Cancer was constructed as a silent and deadly disease. It was seen as the danger within, a malign agent (Sontag 1979) that strikes with no warning. It was regarded as unpredictable, as Patricia said:

> You know, the perfect thing with a cancer is actually when it starts to transport the stuff round your body, and how do you know whether the [breast] lump that you've got is going to be one that's going to move quickly, or one that you can, say, hang around for? You just don't know.

On the other hand, it was also seen as predictable to the extent that, with the exception of Victoria, all thought that if their bodies were left unchecked they would definitely succumb to breast cancer in the future. As Sarah said, 'I wouldn't voluntarily put myself under the knife if I didn't think, well, it was inevitable.' Their experience of genetic counselling appeared to do little to alleviate these women of their fears or change their belief that they would develop cancer. As Tracey said:

> She explained it very well, you know, she said, one in eleven women will get it during their lifetime you're sort of one in five, because you're higher ... It doesn't sound that horrific ... I wanted to hear that, but I still thought, well, I'm still going to get it. Because that's the way I am. ... I've said straight from the start, it's too close to me for me to just brush it off.

All acknowledged that prophylactic surgery was a 'radical' or 'drastic' action, but justified their interest in this procedure on the basis that the elimination of their 'dangerous' organs would remove their fear of developing cancer (Langellier and Sullivan 1998). As Tracey said of her feelings about prophylactic mastectomy: 'Yes, you know, it is radical, but if it takes away that fear, then that can only be a good thing. Because otherwise the fear will get you in the end.'

Nearly all the women believed that their body (pre-surgery) was essentially compromised – that it contained the seeds of its own destruction. They perceived their bodies as potentially out of control and constructed their breasts as biological 'time bombs' which could go off at any moment (Robertson 1998). However, they differed in the extent to which they believed they could control this danger. For the majority, prophylactic surgery – the elimination of the dangerous body parts – was regarded as providing them with the opportunity to prevent cancer occurring and, thus as enabling them to take control of what they perceived as their destiny. Tracey described her reaction the first time she read a magazine article about prophylactic mastectomy for breast cancer risk as follows:

> All of a sudden there was this massive article on these women who had been so proactive and it was just like something like a light coming on you know. What a fantastic idea! ... a great idea you know. That is the most positive thing you can do, you know, then you're not waiting, you're not checking .... I don't want to wait until I get something and then try and do something about it ... I want to make sure I am in control of it.

Similarly, Patricia said that the scars on her reconstructed breasts are a constant reminder of her decision to undergo surgery, a decision she viewed as empowering:

> I like their little scars, because it keeps me in touch with something I've done. It does feel sentimentally a very positive decision, and I like that. I feel, it felt like a way of taking care of myself and actually a way of being taken care of.

Although Victoria was the only woman in this sample who had clinical confirmation of her risk status as a result of genetic testing, she differed from the rest of these women in so far as she was convinced that she would never get cancer; she said she ' ... never at any stage felt that I was going to get cancer, and I still don't now.' Like many of the women in these two studies (Hallowell 1998a and b) she described herself as having an obligation to her family to manage her risk.

Therefore, despite her conviction that she would not develop cancer in the future, she had still felt the need to take control of her body for her family's sake. She talked about surgery as providing her with the opportunity to contain her residual risk, or limit the damage that cancer could inflict upon her body and her family life (cf. Kavanagh and Broom 1998):

> And I don't feel like I'm a cancerous person. I know I've got this gene, but it might not activate. It could lay dormant for ever. And now, if it does, it's got nowhere to go. It can't do much damage. And if I do get breast cancer, it will be here or wherever, and they'll be able to treat it, and it can't spread because there's nowhere, you know.

In contrast, Mandy and Sue were less convinced that surgery would enable them to regain control of their bodies. They did not believe that the removal of their breasts would remove the threat of cancer, for they perceived their bodies as ultimately uncontrollable. As Sue said about cancer, 'sometimes I think there's no getting away from it'. These women questioned the benefits of undergoing surgery and reasoned that even if they underwent prophylactic mastectomy the cancer would either develop in the remaining breast tissue (Sue), or elsewhere in the body. As Mandy said:

> I could have both breasts cut off, and then develop cancer of the ovaries or cancer of the colon or cancer of something else. And you could go on forever in a sense trying to prevent on the basis of not entirely a 100 per cent clear knowledge.

But despite their scepticism both Mandy and Sue were willing to undergo prophylactic surgery because both acknowledged that they had a responsibility to their families to take whatever steps were necessary to reduce their risk. Indeed, they said that they would not hesitate to proceed with prophylactic surgery if they had a positive mutation test result.

In constructing their bodies as bodies 'out of control' and surgery as enabling them to regain control of their body, it could be argued that these women, like those described by Kavanagh and Broom (1998) and Martin (1989), implicitly disassociate the body from the self. The dangerous body in these accounts, like the body of biomedicine, is conceived of as an object that can be manipulated and rendered safe by the disposal of the dangerous parts – their breasts. The removal of these body parts is seen as not only enabling them to eradicate their fear of developing cancer, but as ensuring their survival. However, in reality things are not so straightforward, for, as the next section will demonstrate, although all these women were prepared to manipulate their body in an effort to control what they perceived as its inherent dangers, they also viewed surgery as potentially problematic; they perceived prophylactic mastectomy as a threat to their bodily integrity which could have negative repercussions for their femininity, and therefore, their self-identity.

Dangerous Bodies = Feminine Bodies

> ... to experience oneself and be experienced by others as a woman is to take up a particular bodily identity ... (Shildrick 1997: 48)

According to Sandra Lee Bartky (1990) gendered bodies are produced and maintained as the result of disciplinary practices. She argues that these practices are part of the process by which the 'ideal body of femininity – and hence the feminine body-subject – is constructed' (p. 71). Discipline (for example, dieting, plastic surgery, deportment, using make-up, etc.) results in a properly feminine body, a body that is a particular shape or size, moves in a particular way (Young 1990) and is ornamented or adorned in a particular way. The undisciplined body, the body that is, for example, the wrong shape – is seen as deficient – not properly feminine. Because the disciplinary practices which produce the feminine body are 'institutionally unbounded and all pervasive in western society' (p. 77), Bartky argues that the production of femininity appears to be not only voluntary, but natural. Furthermore, although she observes that these disciplinary practices are disempowering for women in general, in so far as feminine bodies are produced as objects for the male gaze, she also recognizes that discipline can lead to the development of individual powers to the extent that engaging in these practices provides individuals with a 'secure sense of identity' (p. 77) – a feminine identity. Thus, according to this point of view, although gender appears to be naturally inscribed upon the body, the gendered body is socially constructed and actively managed. Moreover, the practice of maintaining or managing the properly feminine body has implications for the self, in the sense that managing the body entails managing the self (Giddens

1991). To be a woman is to have a particular embodied identity.

When voicing their misgivings about prophylactic surgery many women drew upon discourses about the 'naturally' *feminine* body, frequently echoing two ideas in Bartky's analysis: first, that the production and maintenance of a feminine body is perceived and experienced as natural; and, second, that the possession of a properly feminine body is important for women's sense of identity. Thus, according to all the women who took part in this study, one's femininity is, at least in part, dependent upon having a particular type of body – a body with breasts. Breasts were frequently described as 'womanly bits' and removing them was perceived as a threat to one's feminine bodily identity – one's femininity. As Patricia said about her mastectomy: 'It felt very threatening to be a woman with no breasts, it really did I think, before I had it done.'

The appearance of the body was privileged in many of these accounts. Thus, prophylactic mastectomy was described as compromising the feminine body in a profound manner because it results in perceptible changes to the body. A recurrent theme in these interviews was that breasts publicly display one's femininity – having breasts made one look like a 'natural' woman. Having your breasts surgically removed was described as 'radical' because it is unavoidably public. According to these women, the mastectomized body looks different, it is 'unnatural' and therefore, no longer feminine.

These women frequently constructed their breasts as objects for the male gaze (Young 1990; Bartky 1990). For example, Patricia observed:

I think there's also a society thing of the way a woman's body is perceived, and I don't think men are immune from that. And the way women are looked at, like a physical thing, and the breasts are a very important part of that.

However, it wasn't just the fact that their bodies might look different to others following surgery that worried them, for they did not just regard their breasts as things-for-others. Mastectomy was seen as threatening one's identity, the perception of oneself as a 'natural' woman. Many women said their breasts were fundamental to their self-perception, describing themselves, for example, as busty or flat-chested, and thus mastectomy constituted a threat to self-identity. As Sue said, breasts, unlike the uterus and ovaries, are 'part of your womanhood' because 'when you're getting dressed in the morning, when you walk down the street, and you're trying nice clothes on, you've got your breasts there to form your shape, sort of thing ... '

Some women said that it had taken a long time for them to become comfortable with the fact that their body differed from representations of the idealized female body and that overcoming the fact that they did not have a 'perfect' body had meant that they had developed a special relationship with their breasts – they defined their uniqueness. As Sarah said, when talking about reconstructive surgery:

> I don't have a great big pair of boobs that I kind of like show off, because I haven't – but, you know, I quite like what I've got, and to have something in their place, yes, I think every woman would rather than not, basically. I suppose it's a natural –

Clearly, when making a decision about the management of their genetic risk these women are faced with a dilemma, for if they take control of their dangerous bodies and dispose of the dangerous parts, then they expose themselves to other dangers – the loss of a particular embodied identity – they will no longer be 'natural' women. Consequently, most of these women said they would only consider undergoing mastectomy in conjunction with breast reconstruction. For some, prophylactic mastectomy was perceived as providing them with the opportunity to improve their body. Subsequent reconstruction meant that they could have their bodies altered so that they approximated more closely the idealized feminine body they had always desired; as Sarah said, 'Yes, I mean it would be great if they could give me 36Ds instead ... ' Similarly, Victoria described how she had felt before her operation:

> I was looking forward to the boob job. As I said, I was a 34AA, breastfed three children, two little empty sacks – you know? And hated, always hated my boobs, always wanted a boob job. Would never have had one, but always wanted one. I thought, 'Well, here's my chance!'

Although reconstructive surgery offered some of these women the promise of an enhanced or more normalized femininity (Bartky 1990; Young 1990; Lee 1997), all those who considered reconstruction said that their real motivation for undergoing this procedure was that they wanted to still look like a woman post-surgery (cf. Davis 1995). As Neill et al. (1998) have observed, breast reconstruction is frequently perceived as a way of achieving normality following therapeutic mastectomy. The women who took part in this study similarly regarded reconstructive surgery as a way of maintaining their 'natural' feminine bodily identity, as preserving their femininity. Sarah explained why she would opt for a reconstruction if she underwent mastectomy as follows:

> Basically, because I want to be able to go out and go on holidays and wear swimsuits and T-shirts and – I'm not a particularly vain person, you know, I'm not – I suppose – I'm not really a vain person. But ... I just think it would make me feel better to have boobs rather than not. I think that's a pretty – I would imagine that's a natural thing for anybody.

In many cases reconstruction was not only motivated by the need to appear 'natural' to themselves,[1] but also to appear 'natural' in the eyes of others, particularly their sexual partners. Despite reassurance from their partners that the relationship would not be affected by mastectomy, they were worried that they would be less desirable to their sexual partners following mastectomy if they did not have reconstruction. For example, Sue when reflecting upon her potential reactions to mastectomy said:

> ... I think I'd be more bothered about what my partner thought of me without breasts .... And I just think, what if I have – you know? – nothing there and ugly scars and ... ? But then, what's it matter, if you're alive? I can think like that, but then when it comes to putting it into action, it's – it's different.

But although reconstructive surgery was seen as potentially enabling one to maintain one's femininity, it was also described as problematic. All the women were aware of the risks associated with silicon implants and worried that the implants themselves would compromise their bodily integrity. As Mandy, the only woman who was adamant that she would not have reconstructive surgery because of her concerns about the risks associated with silicon implants, said:

> I suspect the silicon implants are not as successful as people make out, that there are all kinds of problems, and I don't think I want to walk round with plastic inside me and all that, you know, it doesn't appeal to me at all.

However, with this one exception, all the women regarded the risks associated with reconstruction as less important than the perceived benefits, i.e. the production or preservation of a feminine-looking body.

Discourses normalize bodies. They set the boundaries of what it is for a body to be feminine or to be at risk. The problem for these women is that their bodily identity is ultimately compromised, for those body parts which society constructs as feminine are isomorphic with those body parts which they construct as dangerous. Consequently, prophylactic surgery presents these women with a dilemma, for if they attempt to manage the dangers inherent within their bodies by removing their breasts they will compromise their feminine bodily identity – they will no longer be a 'natural' woman. As was noted above, most of these women perceived reconstructive surgery as enabling them to resolve the tensions generated by these competing discourses, presenting them with the possibility of managing a life-threatening risk whilst maintaining a feminine bodily shape following mastectomy. This option is not, however, without risk, as all the women were aware.

At the time of these interviews Tracey, Sue, Sarah and Mandy were still undecided about whether they should pursue prophylactic surgery. They were unwilling to disrupt the boundaries of the feminine body by undergoing mastectomy and also unsure about exposing themselves to the risks associated with breast reconstruction. Thus, they had reached what they perceived as a compromise with regard to their risk management, opting to continue with annual breast screening for the present. Although screening potentially exposes their healthy bodies to radiation or unnecessary exploratory operations, these women regarded the risks associated with bodily surveillance as preferable to the disruption of their femininity and bodily integrity which would result from surgery.

Patricia and Victoria, on the other hand, said that they had undergone surgery because they were unconvinced of the benefits of breast screening. They both expressed a large degree of scepticism about the ability of mammography to detect a cancer in the early stages. Victoria said that she had an obligation to her family to do all she could to manage her risk and ensure her survival, no matter what the consequences were to herself. Patricia said she had not been prepared to sacrifice her life in order to maintain her bodily integrity. But although both women said they had been prepared to undergo mastectomy in order that they might contain their risk of breast cancer, they had not been prepared to sacrifice their femininity; thus, both had undergone reconstructive surgery. None the less, as the next section will demonstrate, both experienced their femininity as essentially compromised by surgery, in ways they had not foreseen.

Reconstructed bodies = unnatural bodies

> To have a body felt to be 'feminine' ... is in most cases crucial to a woman's sense of herself as female ... To possess such a body may also be essential to her sense of herself as a sexually desiring and desirable subject.
>
> (Bartky 1990: 77)

Kent (1998) observes that surgery 'disrupts and penetrates the boundaries of the physical body, undermining bodily integrity' (p. 3). She notes that recovery from plastic surgery requires that the individual engages in *'boundary work,* in re-negotiating the significance of her bodily shape and re-constructing identity' (p. 3, emphasis in the original). Both Victoria and Patricia described their experience of surgery as involving this kind of 'boundary work'. They reported that they had found it very hard to come to terms with their new bodies, and ultimately experienced the loss of their breasts as compromising their femininity in a profound manner.

Victoria and Patricia described their new breasts as 'firmer', 'upright' and 'looking good'. Although one of Patricia's nipples was 'in a strange place' and Victoria had lost a nipple after the operation and also had what she described as a 'strange concavey bit' on the side of her chest, both said their reconstructed breasts were more aesthetically pleasing than the ones they had removed, they approximated a more idealized or normalized shape (Young 1990; Lee 1997). Both women revelled in the fact that they no longer needed to wear a bra, and said they felt they looked better in their clothes and could now wear clothes that they would not have worn before the reconstruction. However, although they acknowledged that they still looked like a woman, indeed, that they *looked* more feminine than before the surgery, they both described themselves as feeling 'incomplete' or 'unnatural'.

Iris Young (1990) observes that the look of the breasts is privileged within Western society, in so far as the dominant (phallocentric) discourses objectify breasts as things to be looked at – as objects for the male gaze. She argues that this view of the breasts contrasts with that held by women who, from their position as feminine subjects, consider the feeling and sensitivity of their breasts as much more important than their physical appearance. This point of view was echoed by both Victoria and Patricia who described the lack of feeling and sensitivity in their reconstructed breasts as compromising their femininity. Both women talked at great length about the ways in which their reconstructed breasts felt different. Patricia described the loss of sensitivity in her breasts as causing her great sadness:

> What did I feel I had lost? Um ... a lot of my femininity. A part of my body. My breasts to me were a very important part of my body ... – just the feel of my breasts, not sexually but just against my dress you know, like that was very very big ... it's a physical ... It's a sadness that there isn't that very intense physical pleasure available to me any more, that kind of intense physical – and the less intense is just the feel of the skin on my breasts that just felt nice but particularly sensitive, not particularly sexual but just nicely sensitive which was like a soft womanly part of me, missing that.

Both Patricia and Victoria described the changes in feeling in their breasts as having profound effects on their sexuality. Patricia said that before she underwent surgery she had felt that her sexuality had been threatened, owing to her anxiety that either she or her partner would find a breast lump during sex. Although this threat had dissipated since operation, she still felt that her sexuality was irrevocably compromised by the loss of sensation in her nipples, and she experienced this loss of sensitivity as an explicit threat to her femininity.

> ... sexually it's an enormous difference to me. And it's not that I can't have sexual satisfaction without that [nipple] stimulation, but it's – that stimulation does matter, and it's somehow more than that. It's about part of myself as a woman, to express myself sexually.

Victoria, was also upset about the lack of feeling in her reconstructed breasts and talked about how this had negatively affected her libido. She described herself as needing to renegotiate the boundaries of her body, as having to relearn what it feels like to have her new breasts touched:

I don't like it if my husband touches them. . . . I don't know he's touching them. And I hate that. I look round and he'll like have his hand there or something, and – which isn't very often, believe me. He also knows that I'm a bit funny with my boobs. Um . . . I don't like the fact that I can't feel it. But the feeling is – it is getting a bit better, a bit different. But I don't think they'll ever feel – you see, I was told I would lose a little bit of sensation. I wasn't told they'd be dead. You see, I wasn't really told the truth.

In addition, she talked about how she had to learn that her breasts now moved in a different way. On the positive side, their firmness meant that her breasts 'looked good' and gave her a better shape. However, on the negative side, their lack of manoeuvrability was experienced as uncomfortable, and as restricting the movements of her body more generally.

Even now they're uncomfortable. You know, you can't do certain things. Like if you're lying in bed on your side, you and your husband, and you want a cuddle, it's really uncomfortable for me. . . . your boobs, they're like floppy. And when you go on your side like that [gestures], they'll go down and they'll get comfy in there [gestures]. Whereas mine are solid, they don't manoeuvre that much, you know. If I go down on my side, they're like blocks there.

The fact that their breasts looked different, moved differently, felt different to their touch, were less sensitive and were no longer sexually responsive were not the only things that Victoria and Patricia had to get used to, for what also worried them was that their breasts felt different to others. The boundaries of their bodies had been transgressed by the insertion of an alien substance which not only made their breasts feel different to themselves, but marked them out as different to others. They were very conscious of the fact that their breasts were no longer soft and yielding to other people's touch and were aware that as far as others were concerned their breasts felt unnatural – they were 'solid' or like 'blocks'. Thus, they described their breasts as 'a buffer' between them and other people. As Victoria said:

If I knock you, if I walk by you, and my boob gets caught, it's like there's a buffer there, and I think, 'I wonder what she just felt? Do I feel normal?' You know, when people cuddle me, I sort of pull back a bit now, because I don't like my boobs to touch them. A few close people, I'll say, 'What does it feel like when you cuddle me?' But I don't know if they tell me the truth.

And Patricia:

> ... I've had a lot of hugs from women lately, and they come up and I can feel their breasts against mine, and mine feel different. And with children I'm aware of that, you know, the bigger ones, you know, and you give them a hug and you're aware, and my breasts feel very different. They're not so soft. And that's just sad.

Young (1990) argues that the sense of touch is important because it is reciprocal – at one and the same time it is active and passive. In touching another, one simultaneously touches and is touched. In this sense touching, in contrast to looking, blurs the boundaries between self and other, subject and object. In losing their breasts, what Victoria and Patricia lost was the ability to touch others and to be touched. The immediacy of feeling they had previously experienced when their breasts were touched by or touched others was now experienced at second-hand. Thus, by creating a physical barrier between them and the rest of the world, their reconstructed breasts constructed a psychological barrier which they had to overcome. Patricia in particular worried that this 'difference' would deter others from having a sexual relationship with her:

> I'm beginning to be very aware that if I have a new relationship, I'm not as I seem. Physically I'm not as I seem. And I'm not sure how to handle that, and there's an obvious difference in somebody who is like physically complete, and basically in some sense I'm not physically complete. ... I sort of realise that even the most loving person is going to have like wants and desires, and for a partner to be, oh I don't know what's the – just not completely natural I suppose in my sexual perception, it is a big thing.

As Young (1990) observes, breasts are not only objects for male desire, but are intrinsically bound up with feminine subjectivity. Breasts do not just make bodies look feminine; having breasts also makes one feel like a woman. The removal of their natural breasts and the subsequent loss of feeling they experienced in their reconstructed breasts meant that although Victoria and Patricia measured up well against the normalizing gaze – they looked feminine – they did not experience their body as a feminine body. Throughout these accounts these women constructed their reconstructed breasts as 'other'. Although their bodies looked 'properly' feminine, they felt incomplete. They perceived their bodies as deficient – as unnatural – and therefore, regarded surgery as compromising their femininity. Thus, managing their risk of breast cancer not only necessitated that they come to terms with a new body shape, or way of physically being-in-the-world, as Victoria said, 'I'm just starting to now like them [breasts] a little bit. I hated them. I hated them', but also required that they underwent a process of reconstructing their identity. Prophylactic mastectomy plus reconstruction resulted in the creation of a new feminine identity for these women – they perceived themselves as 'incomplete' or not fully 'natural' women. Victoria described herself as: 'coming through it now. It took its time. I mean I did hit rock bottom ... it's taken its time. And I had to learn to – to like myself again.' Similarly, Patricia said that learning to live with her new breasts – the physical reconstruction of her body – had required an extensive period of psychological reconstruction, which was still ongoing two years after surgery:

> ... in order to help IVF I've had my tubes clipped, and so they are now cut away from my uterus, and it's like, you know, what is left of my femininity? You know? My reproductive organs are just in a complete state and I don't have my breasts. I mean I have to say also that as I grow stronger in a sense of self, that has less impact. I think it's very dependent on, you know, your strength of self. But it is still there. It is still there and it needs fixing.

But despite the negative implications of this form of risk management for their self-identity, neither woman regretted her decision to undergo surgery. They regarded mastectomy as removing a life-threatening risk; as Patricia said 'two years ago, well ten years ago, I'd have told you I'd be dead, I'd have cancer – I expected to have cancer by 45. I just thought that my body was diseased completely. I just don't feel that now.' Both women viewed the disruption of their femininity, and the subsequent boundary work they had to engage in, as a price worth paying to control the dangers within their bodies, as Patricia said: 'My life is more precious to me, you know, than part of my femininity or my sexuality which I can learn to have in other ways.' From Victoria's point of view, although surgery had compromised her feminine bodily identity, it had also enabled her to fulfil her obligations of care and thus, preserve her identity as carer, as a self-in-relation.

Managing the Body = Managing the Self

This chapter suggests that the role played by the breasts in the construction of femininity has profound implications for the ways in which women manage their risk of breast cancer. The analysis of women's accounts of their experiences indicated that living with and managing the risk of breast cancer appears to be fraught with contradictions. On the one hand, these accounts revealed a certain degree of fragmentation between body and self (cf. Kavanagh and Broom 1998). These women constructed their breasts as other, as 'dangerous objects' which threatened their very existence. According to this point of view, prophylactic surgery – the removal of their dangerous body parts – was conceived as providing them with the means to regain control of the body and therefore, as protecting the self.

On the other hand, there was evidence that these women perceived the self as necessarily embodied (Giddens 1991), for although they constructed their bodies as out of control (cf. Martin 1989), they did not perceive their breasts as body parts that can be disposed of without implications for self-identity. All the women in this study constructed their breasts as internally related to their femininity – to be a woman is to be breasted and vice versa. Accordingly, managing their risk of breast cancer by removing their breasts was seen as a potential threat to their femininity. Thus, it can be argued that the degree of fragmentation between self and body documented by Kavanagh and Broom (1998) was not evident in these accounts. On the contrary, these accounts revealed that bodily identity and integrity is important for their sense of self-identity, in so far as the body parts implicated in this instance – the breasts – were constructed as internally related to gender identity.

These accounts also revealed that the role played by the body in the construction of gender identity is not straightforward. Prior to surgery these women privileged the look of their breasts in the maintenance of their femininity. Like Bartky (1990) they talked about how their sense of identity was dependent upon their possessing a properly 'feminine' body – looking like a woman. Thus, they described their femininity as being dependent upon maintaining a particular bodily shape – having breasts. Mastectomy was, therefore, viewed as a threat to their femininity in so far as it results in a deficient body – a body that is no longer feminine. For those who had not yet undergone surgery, the materiality of the body, whether it is composed of flesh or silicon, was seen as less important than having a body that looks feminine. Therefore, despite the fact that it is a risky procedure, breast reconstruction was perceived by many of these women as providing them with a way in which they could resolve the tensions generated by the competing discourses of the naturally feminine body and the dangerous body. Reconstructive surgery produces normalized bodies – feminine-looking bodies – and thus was perceived as enabling one to maintain one's femininity following mastectomy.

However, the women who had subjected their bodies to this form of discipline told a different story. For these women the fact that the look of their reconstructed breasts approached the normalized ideal to a greater extent than before was less important for their feminine bodily identity than the loss of sensitivity and feeling in their breasts they experienced post-surgery. Although they regarded themselves as looking like 'natural' women following reconstructive surgery, they did not experience themselves as such. These women privileged the feeling of their breasts in the maintenance of their femininity (Young 1990), describing their femininity, at least in part, as grounded within the materiality of their bodies. As far as they were concerned, the materiality of their body, how it felt to themselves and others, was much more important than how it looked; consequently, they felt that their femininity had been compromised by their efforts to maintain a normalized feminine-looking body.

Although these accounts would appear to provide support for Bartky's analysis, they also suggest that the role of the body in the construction of gender identity is more complex than she intimates. In particular, the accounts of women who had undergone breast reconstruction suggest that femininity is not just dependent upon managing one's body so it complies with the standards of bodily acceptability – it looks feminine – but that it is also dependent upon experiencing a particular type of material embodiment. As far as these women were concerned, although they were aware that they appeared feminine, this was not how they felt. They experienced their bodies as different, and this had implications for their sense of identity.

Thus, it can be argued that this analysis indicates that the materiality of the body is also implicated in the construction of gender identity. In making this claim I am not, however, adopting an essentialist line on the development of gender identity, nor subscribing to the view that gender differences are determined by biological sex differences, i.e. that gender is a natural category. What I am suggesting is that bodies are not neutral material upon which gender is inscribed (cf. Gatens 1996; Grosz 1994) , but rather that the materiality of the body – the way it is configured or composed – has implications for the social construction of gendered bodies. In other words, gender is inscribed on bodies which have a particular structure, and the experience of gendered embodiment is affected by the material body. This does not mean that the way in which the material body affects the experience of gendered embodiment is given a priori (Gatens 1994; Grosz 1996),[2] i.e. that the material body determines gendered embodiment, but rather that material bodies afford certain possibilities which may or may not play a role in the construction of masculine and feminine bodies. Thus, the production and maintenance of a feminine body, as described by Bartky, is not just dependent on disciplinary practices *per se*, but on disciplinary practices working on a particular type of material substrate, namely, a material body that is configured in a certain way. According to this point of view, changing the material configuration or composition of the body, as in this case by removing or replacing the breast tissue, will have repercussions for gender identity.

In conclusion, this chapter has argued that the geneticization of breast cancer has profound implications for women who have a family history of this disease. It not only exposes them to medical interventions which may have iatrogenic consequences and potentially affects their emotional well-being, but it also affects the way in which they think about their bodies and, by implication, their sense of self-identity. The analysis outlined above suggests that women who are identified as at risk of hereditary breast cancer have an ambivalent relationship with their bodies. On the one hand, their breasts provide them with the secure sense of identity, on the other, they expose them to risk and uncertainty. Their bodies afford a particular type of existence within the world yet at the same time they threaten this existence. Finally, it can be argued that this research has implications for the way in which we think about the social construction of gendered bodies in our society. It suggests that gender identity is not only dependent on having a body that is disciplined to appear feminine, but is also dependent upon being a body, i.e. experiencing a particular type of material embodiment.

Acknowledgements

I would like to thank all of the women who took part in this research, Professor B.A.J. Ponder and Dr C. Eng who provided access to their clinics, The Steering Committee of the UKCCCR Familial Ovarian Cancer Register, Carole Pye, Ginny Morrow and Shelley Day Sclater who made many helpful comments about earlier drafts of this manuscript, Helen Statham and Frances Murton. Study 1 was funded by the Medical Research Council Grant No. 303315 awarded to J.M. Green and M.P.M. Richards. The familial cancer clinic was supported by grants from the Cancer Research Campaign [CRC] to B.A.J. Ponder. Study 2 was funded by WellBeing (RCOG) in a grant awarded to the author. An earlier version of this paper was presented at the annual BSA conference 'Making Sense of the Body' in Edinburgh in April 1998.

*   *   *

In May 1998 one of my oldest and closest friends had a therapeutic mastectomy to treat a recurrence of breast cancer. We have talked about this a lot over the past few months, and these discussions have undoubtedly influenced the way I have approached this analysis. Without Fiona this paper would have been entirely different. I might not have got so mad and upset whilst I was writing, or I might have thought that there was a neat and tidy solution to some of these questions. I now know there is not. Whilst I was writing this chapter Fiona was never far from my mind, so I now dedicate it to her, with love.

Notes

1 See Davis (1995) who argues that women who undergo cosmetic surgery insist that this is something they do for themselves not for other people within their lives. She observes the women in her study who had cosmetic surgery on their faces or breasts underwent these procedures because they were uncomfortable with their bodies, not because they wanted to be 'more beautiful'. Cosmetic surgery offered them the opportunity to feel 'normal', 'ordinary' and like others (p. 161). Thus, she concludes that although cosmetic surgery presents women with a dilemma, it can also be seen as empowering for some women because it allows them to renegotiate their relationship with their bodies and ultimately enables them to become 'embodied subjects'.

2 Despite the fact that both Gatens and Grosz acknowledge the existence of

material sex differences they do not regard the material body as given, for they observe that biological differences do not have a fixed significance independently of the cultural context in which they are apprehended, although Gatens argues that 'some bodily experiences and events ... are likely in all social structures to be privileged sites of significance' (p. 5).

References

Bartky, S.L. *Femininity and Domination: Studies in the Phenomenology of Oppression* (New York: Routledge 1990).

Cooper, C. and E. Dennison. 'Do Silicone Breast Implants Cause Connective Tissue Disease?' *British Medical Journal,* 316 (1998) pp. 403–4.

Davis, K. *Reshaping the Female Body: The Dilemma of Cosmetic Surgery* (New York and London: Routledge 1995).

Den Otter, W., T.E. Merchant, D. Beijerinck and J.W. Kotten. 'Breast Cancer Induction Due to Mammographic Screening in Hereditarily Affected Women'. *Anticancer Research,* 16 (1996) pp. 3173–6.

Douglas, M. *Risk and Blame: Essays in Cultural Theory.* (London: Routledge 1992).

Douglas, M. and A. Wildavsky, *Risk and Culture* (Berkeley University of California Press 1982).

Easton, D.F., D. Ford, D.T. Bishop and the Breast Cancer Linkage Consortium. 'Breast and Ovarian Cancer Incidence in BRCA1 Mutation Carriers'. *American Journal of Human Genetics,* 56 (1995) pp. 265–71.

Foucault, M. 'On the Genealogy of Ethics: An Overview of Work in Progress'. In P. Rabinow, ed. *The Foucault Reader.* (Harmondsworth: Penguin 1984) pp. 340–72.

Gatens, M. *Imaginary Bodies: Ethics, Power and Corporeality* (London: Routledge 1996).

Grosz, E. *Volatile Bodies: Towards a Corporeal Feminism* (Bloomington and Indianapolis: Indiana University Press, 1994).

Giddens, A. *Modernity and Self Identity: The Self and Society in the Late Modern Age* (Cambridge: Polity Press, 1991).

Hallowell, N. 'Doing the Right Thing: Genetic Risk and Responsibility'. Mimeo, Centre for Family Research, University of Cambridge (1998a).

Hallowell, N. 'Risk Management Following Genetic Testing: Women's Information Needs'. Paper presented at the Fifth International Meeting on the Psychosocial Aspects of Genetic Testing for Hereditary Breast and/or Ovarian Cancer. Leuven, 29–30 June (1998b).

Hartmann, L., R. Jenkins, D. Schaid and P. Yang. 'Prophylactic Mastectomy: Preliminary Retrospective Cohort Analysis'. *Proceedings of the American Association for Cancer Research,* 38 (1997) p. 168.

Illich, I. *Medical Nemesis: The Expropriation of Health* (London: Calder & Boyars 1975).

Jofesson, D. 'High Risk of False Positives with Breast Screening'. *British Medical Journal* 316 (1998) pp. 1261–2.

Kash, K., J.C. Holland, M.S. Halper and D.G. Miller. 'Psychological Distress and Surveillance Behaviours of Women with a Family History of Breast Cancer'.

Journal of the National Cancer Institute 84 (1991) pp. 24–30.

Kavanagh, A.M. and D.H. Broom. 'Embodied Risk: My Body, Myself?' *Social Science and Medicine* 46 (1998) pp. 437–44.

Kent, J. 'Boundary Work: Living With a New Shape'. Paper presented at the British Sociological Association Conference 'Making Sense of the Body: Research and Practice', Edinburgh, 6–9 April (1998).

Langelleir K.M. and C.F. Sullivan, 'Breast Talk in Breast Cancer Narratives'. *Qualitative Health Research* 8 (1998) pp. 76–94.

Lee, J. 'Never Innocent: Breasted Experience in Women's Bodily Narratives of Puberty', *Feminism and Psychology* 7 (1997) pp. 453–74.

Lerman C. and M. Schwartz. 'Adherence and Psychological Adjustment among Women at High Risk for Breast Cancer'. *Breast Cancer Research and Treatment* 28 (1993) pp. 145–55.

Lippman, A. 'Led (Astray) by Genetic Maps: The Cartography of the Human Genome and Healthcare', *Social Science & Medicine* 35 (1992) pp. 1469–76.

Martin, E. *The Woman in the Body* (Milton Keynes: Open University Press 1989).

Miki, J., J. Swensen, D. Shattuck-Eidens et al., 'A Strong Candidate for the Breast Ovarian Cancer Susceptibility Gene BRCA1', *Science* 266 (1994) pp. 66–71.

Muhr, T. *Atlas-ti: Computer Aided Text Interpretation and Theory Building* (Berlin, 1994).

Neugut A.I. and J.S. Jacobson. 'The Limitations of Breast Cancer Screening for First Degree Relatives of Breast Cancer Patients'. *American Journal of Public Health* 85 (1995) pp. 832–4.

Neill, K.M., N. Armstrong and C.B. Burnett. 'Choosing Reconstruction after Mastectomy: A Qualitative Analysis'. *Oncology Nursing Forum* 25 (1998) pp. 743–50.

Nuffield Council on Bioethics. *Genetic Screening: Ethical Issues* (London: The Nuffield Council 1993).

Robertson, A. 'Our Bodies, Our Enemies: Women's Perceptions of Risk of Breast Cancer'. Paper presented at the British Sociological Association Conference 'Making Sense of the Body: Research and Practice', Edinburgh, 6–9th April (1998).

Schrag, D., K.M. Kuntz, J. Garber and J.C. Weeks. 'Decision Analysis-Effects of Prophylactic Mastectomy and Oophorectomy on Life Expectancy among Women with *BRCA1* or *BRCA2* Mutations'. *New England Journal of Medicine,* 336 (1997) pp. 1465–71.

Shildrick, M. *Leaky Bodies and Boundaries: Feminism, Postmodernism and (Bio)ethics* (London: Routledge 1997).

Sontag, S. *Illness as a Metaphor* (Harmondsworth: Penguin 1979).

Stacey, J. *Teratologies: a Cultural Study of Cancer* (London: Routledge 1997).

Stephanek, M.E., K.J. Helzlsouer, P.M. Wilcox and F. Houn. 'Predictors of and Satisfaction with Bilateral Prophylactic Mastectomy'. *Preventative Medicine* 24 (1995) pp. 412–19.

Tonin, P., P. Ghadirian, C. Phelan et al. 'A Large Multisite Cancer Family is Linked to BRCA2'. *Journal of Medical Genetics* 32 (1995) pp. 982–4.

Wooster, R., S. Neuhausen, J. Mangion et al. 'Localisation of a Breast Cancer Susceptibility Gene (BRCA2) to Chromosome 13q by Linkage Analysis'. *Science* 265 (1994) pp. 2088–90.

Young, I.M. *Throwing Like a Girl and Other Feminist Philosophy and Social Theory* (Bloomington and Indianapolis: Indiana University Press 1990).

Ziegler L.D. and S.S. Kroll. 'Primary Breast Cancer after Prophylactic Mastectomy'. *American Journal of Clinical Oncology* 14 (1991) pp. 451–4.

Zola, I.K. 'Medicine as an Institution of Social Control'. *Sociological Review* 20 (1972) pp. 487–504.

7

Assessing Breast Cancer: Risk, Science and Environmental Activism in an 'At Risk' Community

Jennifer Fishman

Debates about potential links between breast cancer and the environment emerge as one of the sites where 'at risk' individuals have expressed resistance and distrust of techno-industries and their perceived toxic products. As a result, breast cancer has become a 'controversial' illness, in that hypotheses about causal explanations proliferate, with environmental toxins particularly often identified as a potential cause of the disease. Individuals who bear the burden of health risks produced by techno-industries have at times reacted with resistance to and distrust of the technologies themselves, the social institutions that produce them, and the science of risk assessment developed to evaluate them. Often these individuals develop resistance in response to their own knowledge of or experiences with illnesses that they believe are due at least in part to techno-industrial, environmental toxins present in their local communities. Although some scientific 'experts' may perceive these beliefs as an irrational distrust of scientific and governmental institutions, they can also be read as subversive resistance to risk management's claims of innocent, 'value-free' risk assessment projects.

Risk assessment science itself comes under unique criticism by activists concerned with breast cancer, in that attaining risk information for cancer in general is notoriously problematic. Thus, risk assessment science comes to be viewed as perpetually uncertain, incomplete and inadequate and this is especially true when it comes to linking cancer and the environment. These inadequacies are, however, seldom acknowledged by the risk 'experts' who rely on such scientific knowledge to generate definitive findings about risk factors and who is deemed 'at risk,' which in turn directly influence health policy, funding and research decisions.

This chapter focuses on a particular example of the processes of resistance and reconstruction of risk assessment through an analysis of the experiences and activities of an 'at risk' community. Bayview Hunters Point is primarily an African-American district in the corner of San Francisco that bears a heavy burden of toxic waste sites and hazardous materials sites. Bayview Hunters Point also has the second highest age-adjusted rates of breast cancer among all districts in San Francisco (Aragon and Grumbach 1997), and has twice the number of breast cancer cases among women under fifty than would be expected for that age group (San Francisco Chronicle Staff 1995). A task force was developed in the community to assess the environmental and health effects in this neighbourhood, and in particular the possible effects of the environment on breast cancer rates. Community residents on the task force have, through their activist efforts, insisted on playing a central role at every level of the risk assessment research and the production of scientific risk knowledge. Because of the distrust of the local scientific and governmental institutions that have failed the community in the past, these residents have used their involvement to construct the risk assessment project to reflect their concerns about their community and about the science of risk assessment itself. This analysis will centre on the community activists' constructions of risk assessment *not* as an objective, 'innocent' science, but as one that is deeply influenced by the political, exploitative, elitist and racist practices of the institutions in which it is embedded.

Risk assessment science has become a contested terrain for everyone concerned with issues of environmental risk, especially as it relates to cancer. Although scientific knowledge is often conceived as the product of scientists alone, in the case of risk knowledge, knowledge production has been expropriated by activists and others and placed in a larger social arena. In this larger arena, the core issues of the production of such knowledge and the questions of who is entitled to produce it become intensely problematized. In the case of Bayview Hunters Point, like other similarly situated communities, these questions are closely linked to larger concerns about environmental racism, institutional accountability and identity politics.

The Social Studies of Risk Assessment Science

Embedded in epidemiology, the science of risk assessment uses statistical procedures to calculate a 'relative risk' of a given exposure to a 'dangerous' element, meaning that it determines the risk of a particular health effect (e.g. breast cancer) from exposure to a health hazard based on how much higher that risk is *relative* to what would be expected in an unexposed population. Typically approached as a three-step process, involving hazard identification, dose response evaluation and analysis of exposure, these procedures together result in a quantitative risk assessment (Silbergeld 1991). After the relative risk numbers are produced, the next step is that of risk management, which includes all the processes of judgement and decision-making: the considerations of acceptability, feasibility, equity and economics. Although the US Environmental Protection Agency formally separated the process of risk management from risk assessment in order to delineate the differences between 'hard' science and the policy-making, in recent years this distinction has been challenged, and, more often than not, 'risk management' is placed under the larger umbrella of 'risk assessment' (Perhac 1998). Those who challenge the separation understand that this distinction is in many ways a false one which implies that the risk 'scientists' do not make value judgements of their own throughout the assessment process. Other risk scientists have been engaging in further claims-making activities of their own to reinforce the legitimacy of this scientific knowledge, through rhetoric about its 'objective,' scientific, and therefore, authoritative properties (Abraham and Sheppard 1997).

If we take seriously the claim by academicians and lay publics that risk is socially and culturally constructed (e.g. Beck 1992; Douglas 1992; Freudenburg 1993; Jacobs and Dopkeen 1990; Lambert and Rose 1996; Shrader-Frechette 1991; Wynne 1996), then we must consider the ways in which science and scientific institutions shape and frame their constructions of risk, as a form of scientific knowledge, in certain ways to achieve certain ends. Regardless of what type of risk is being analysed, risk analysts, as positivist scientists, produce what they consider to be an objective assessment of the risk in question. This scientific knowledge, like others, is seen as unproblematic and 'objective', not only because of its quantitative embodiment of risk but also because of the mere fact that the knowledge is located in the authoritative realm of science (Beck 1992; Freudenburg 1993; Wynne 1996). As an outgrowth of modernization and the cultural-political hegemony of scientism, this becomes the dominant discourse of risk (Beck 1992). Understanding risk as something calculable, controllable and therefore preventable reflects some of the fundamental themes of modernity (Prior 1995).

In the postmodern era, dominant risk paradigms are being reconceptualized and re-evaluated. Such critiques stem from both social scientists and lay publics who claim that such risk analyses are not 'innocent' and value-free as risk analysts claim, but are instead embedded in ethical ideas and politics (Douglas 1992; McKechnie 1996; Shrader-Frechette 1991). The normative, universalizing, modernist model of risk makes assumptions not only about people's motivations to act 'rationally', but also more political assumptions about the utility of technology, the moral responsibilities of individuals, what are the best interests of a community and how they might be served, and the role of science in society. The results of such risk analyses, therefore, not only assume how the public should respond to risks, but in many ways decide, in their very formulation, which risks are deemed dangerous or worrisome and which can be safely dismissed. While clearly there are different orders of magnitude in the danger that different objects pose to us, the question that remains is how social agents categorize that which is dangerous (Clarke and Short 1993).

Environmental risk debates not only involve negotiations around what should be done about a particular environmental risk, how it can be 'managed' and what its consequences are, but necessarily involve a negotiation over the very definitions and meanings attached to 'environmental risk'. The politics of the production of risk knowledge has meant that activists and those considered (or who consider themselves) 'at risk' from the environment have wrested the production of this knowledge away from the privileged purview of 'scientists' and have placed it into a social and political arena. Through these claims one's knowledge becomes authoritative and therefore shapes the overlapping scientific and political directions of the issue. The production of scientific knowledge emerges out of *credibility struggles* (Epstein 1996), whereby the interested actors' claims of credibility rest on their believability and authenticity within the social arena. Each of the actors within this arena has an interest in constructing and framing what is meant by environmental risk, and, perhaps even more importantly, *who* has the authority and authenticity to define it. The claims on which 'at risk' community members base their credibility in the arena often lie in sharp contrast to those of the risk 'experts' (Wynne 1996). Where the risk experts depend on the authoritative nature of scientific knowledge, based on fundamental concepts such as objectivity, validity and 'truth', the community activists from Bayview Hunters Point employ very different credibility claims: their claims-making activities centre on issues of trust in governmental institutions, their authenticity as community residents and their political commitments and racial identity.

These environmental health activists represent an example of a local social movement that takes as one of its primary tasks to engage directly with the production of scientific knowledge and the debates that ensue. By engaging the 'experts' in this way, not only do the activists resist the traditional practices of the production of risk knowledge, but they contribute to the reform of the processes themselves, such that *they* become credible 'experts'. Epstein (1996: 13) speaks eloquently to this point:

> Perhaps the most interesting of the social movements that position themselves in relation to science are those which try to stake out some ground on the scientists' own terrain. These activists wrangle with scientists on issues of truth and method. They seek not only to reform science by exerting pressure from the outside but also to perform science by locating themselves on the inside. They question not just the *uses* of science, not just the *control over* science, but sometimes even the very *contents* of science and the *processes* by which it is produced. Most fundamentally, they claim to speak credibly as experts in their own right – as people who know about things scientific and who can partake of this special and powerful discourse of truth. Most intriguingly, they seek to change the ground rules about how the game of science is played. (emphases in original)

Epstein's analysis of these types of social movements is echoed in my analysis of the activities in Bayview Hunters Point, where the environmental health activists resist and reform the risk assessment project, and risk assessment science through contesting various aspects of environmental risk. Their resistance entails contesting how risk science will be used for the community; who has control over the production of this science; what the scientific process will be able to say about the community's health; and the methods by which this scientific knowledge is attained. The contestations located within the 'game of science' position the activists within scientific discourses, and in turn allow them to question the very foundations of the authoritative knowledge status granted to risk assessment.

Bayview Hunters Point – History and Background

I conducted an ethnographic study of the claims-making activities of community residents on a community-based task force in Bayview Hunters Point. Bayview Hunters Point (BVHP) is a district in the southeast area of San Francisco which bears a heavy burden of toxic waste sites, hazardous materials sites, one federal Superfund[1] clean-up site and one California Superfund clean-up site. Once primarily a naval station that housed navy families and provided over 15,000 jobs (Johnson 1995), BVHP has since become a residential neighbourhood. The Hunters Point Naval Shipyard, which closed in 1974, was declared a Federal Superfund Site in 1986.

Approximately 62 per cent of the BVHP population of 28,000 is African-American. Asian American/Pacific Islanders account for another 22 per cent of the population. Whites account for approximately 11 per cent and other minorities account for 6 per cent of the community (Environmental Law and Justice Clinic 1998). More than 30 per cent of the BVHP residents have household incomes below $15,000, as compared to the overall city's percentage of 19 per cent. Forty-six per cent of the community residents have incomes below $25,000 (Environmental Law and Justice Clinic 1998).

Recent research has shown that people of colour are disproportionately exposed to greater environmental risks in both community and occupational settings (Bullard 1983; Robinson 1984; Vaughan and Nordenstam 1991); several studies have found an association between the ethnic make-up of a community and the number of hazardous waste sites in that community (Bullard 1983; Commission for Racial Justice 1987). These findings are validated in San Francisco, where the area of BVHP which has the largest population of African-American residents in the city also contains the largest percentage of contaminated hazardous waste sites of any district in San Francisco. While BVHP makes up less than 5 per cent of the city's population, 30 per cent of the hazardous waste sites currently under investigation by the California Environmental Protection Agency are located in BVHP (Bayview Hunters Point Health and Environmental Task Force 1996). A recent report of the Bayview Hunters Point Health and Environmental Task Force found that there are over 700 hazardous waste material facilities, 325 underground petroleum storage tanks, two power plants and a sewage treatment facility, in addition to the two Superfund clean-up sites in BVHP (Bayview Hunters Point Health and Environmental Task Force 1996).

In 1995, the BVHP Health and Environmental Assessment Task Force was created as a collaborative effort between BVHP neighbourhood residents, the San Francisco Department of Public Health, and other public and private institutions in San Francisco. The original purpose for the creation of the Task Force was to address the issue of building a third power plant in BVHP. This led the Task Force to conduct a community-wide study of the health effects that might in part be attributed to the presence of the large number of industrial plants and storage facilities in BVHP. A community health profile was generated by the Task Force to assess health problems in BVHP. The key findings of this report are that for the period of 1991-2, BVHP had among the highest hospitalization rates for asthma, chronic obstructive pulmonary disease, hypertension, congestive heart failure and diabetes mellitus in all age groups, not only in the City of San Francisco but also in the State of California (Aragon and Grumbach 1997). For the period 1987–93, BVHP had the second highest age-adjusted rates of breast and cervical cancer among districts in San Francisco (Aragon and Grumbach 1997). Another report found that breast cancer rates in BVHP among women under age 50 were double what would be expected (San Francisco Chronicle Staff 1995). Women in Bayview Hunters Point with breast cancer have an 87 per cent higher chance of dying than those who live elsewhere in the city (Aragon and Grumbach 1997).

One of the reasons why the Task Force became concerned with issues of environmental health effects and industrial toxins, and more specifically with issues of environmental racism, is because of the study's findings that rates of breast cancer were disproportionately high among young African-American women in BVHP. One of the most important aspects of this research finding was that it was somewhat unexpected: African-American women in the United States are generally considered at *lesser* risk for breast cancer than their white counterparts. In dominant discourse, breast cancer is considered to be a disease of white middle-class women. The excess number of breast cancer cases in Bayview amongst African-American women means that not only is the risk of breast cancer higher for women in Bayview than for other African-American women in San Francisco, but their risk is also higher than for most *white* women in the city. Because of popular ideas that breast cancer does not affect communities of colour, this fact came as an unwelcome surprise, and moreover became a rallying point around which activists galvanized. Understanding risk in this way has a number of effects on the burgeoning environmental justice movement in BVHP. Because of the high rates of a somewhat unexpected type of cancer in their (black) community, the activists turn to examine the 'environment' in BVHP as the primary culprit. In addition, the activists must contend with other established arenas of breast cancer activism in San Francisco (see Maren Klawiter's chapter in this volume).

Methods

Data Collection

There were two main data collection activities for this project. First, I conducted ongoing participant observation of the Bayview Hunters Point Health and Environmental Assessment Task Force meetings, sub-committee meetings and activities. I attended the general Task Force meetings which meet once a month; these sessions are generally attended by most Task Force members who include BVHP residents, Department of Public Health employees, other local governmental representatives and representatives of public and private health care institutions, and are open to the public. Sub-committees of the Task Force, such as the Breast Cancer Task Force, the Asthma Task Force and the Research Committee, meet weekly to discuss particular issues. Beginning in October 1997 and continuing through April 1998, I attended as many meetings as possible, including all general Task Force meetings, Research Committee meetings and other sub-committee meetings in order to: (a) observe the community-based process of the Task Force as it progresses towards reaching its goals; and (b) analyse how Task Force members discuss and engage with issues about environmental risk, risk assessment research, community involvement, as well as other issues that inevitably arose throughout the project period. Participant observation, also referred to as ethnographic research, consists of entering the social worlds of the participant (Spradley 1980). In this case the social world refers to the events and meetings of the Task Force, as well as other community-based activities and locales. Through in-depth observation and informal interviews and the subsequent recording of these events I collected data in the form of field notes that were then analysed (see below for analysis).

Second, I conducted in-depth qualitative interviews with key informants. I conducted five semi-structured interviews with Task Force members, all of whom are African-Americans. Four of the informants are residents of Bayview Hunters Point, and the fifth considers herself a community representative and advocate and is director of the only health centre in Bayview Hunters Point. Interviews lasted between 50 minutes and one hour and 45 minutes, and were tape-recorded with permission of the informants.

Data Analysis

I analysed the ethnographic data using 'grounded theory'. Grounded theory involves careful reading and coding of the data to generate interpretations and understandings that address the research questions (Hammersley and Atkinson 1996). I began analysis at the outset of data collection to capture key concepts as they emerged, and then was able to integrate concepts into subsequent interviews with other informants. The field notes and transcripts of the audio-taped interviews serve as the data in this project. The text was coded into concepts and sub-concepts based on both the investigator's area of inquiry and also on the concepts that emerged from the data as ones that are significant to the participants (Strauss and Corbin 1990). The conceptual codes were categorized into broader (and narrower) categories and sub-categories. Through this process of 'constant comparison' (Glazer and Strauss 1967) where one code category is compared to the others, an analytic framework was developed.

Authority, Authenticity and Science in BVHP

Throughout my observations and interviews in Bayview Hunters Point, it was apparent that one of the primary sites of contestation for the activists is how risk assessment and other scientific research is to be conducted in their community. Through negotiations over the production of risk knowledge and the identity debates over who it is that gets to produce such knowledge, the community activists engage in claims-making activities that legitimate their role and their authority over matters of local environmental risk. Formerly a concern for risk scientists alone, the process of risk assessment became a negotiated concern for all members of the Task Force, and for community activists in particular. Understanding why risk *science* was chosen as the primary site of contestation leads us to an understanding of how credibility struggles are often waged. Instead of allowing the various 'experts' (e.g. public health epidemiologists, healthcare professionals, healthcare organizations) to claim authority over the problem of environmental risk and breast cancer, thereby dictating how risk will be managed in BVHP, the community activists chose to fight for credibility on the same grounds – that of science. Because of previous negative experiences with scientific and governmental authorities and the detrimental effects of this scientific research, these community members simultaneously understand the important role that scientific assessments can have in the political sphere, yet are deeply distrustful of such research. In other words, this analysis poses the following question: Why are community activists engaging in risk assessment research, a scientific process that they see as historically detrimental and damaging for their community? What is often seen by scientific authorities as an irrational distrust of scientific and governmental institutions can instead be read as a resistance to and *reconstruction* of a science, and of traditional epidemiological studies that have failed and betrayed these residents in the past.

The resistance based on disillusionment and distrust is countered with a reconstruction of the research process by these activists, which focuses on the need for autonomy and independence of the community members to guide the epidemiologic research and to provide programmes for improving the health in the community. The bias that these community members understand to be part of risk assessment science, based on the location of this scientific practice in exploitative, elitist and racist institutions, can, they feel, be rectified through a reconstruction of that science by community members themselves. Through questioning the supposed 'objectivity' of the risk assessment science conducted in BVHP by pointing out the biases of the *experts*, the activists' claims-making carried more weight in the social arena. For it was the activists' claims of authenticity – that only they could know what was 'really' going on in their community – that not only secured their place in the social arena, but gave them leverage in the struggles over credibility.

Institutional Failings

The community activists' critique of the supposedly objective and value-neutral claims of epidemiologic research is based primarily on locating the practice of this science in the governmental and scientific institutions that have failed this community in the past. Previous interactions with these authorities affect their present interactions with those authorities who have come into BVHP to conduct risk assessment research. Perceived discrimination and institutional distrust fuel the scepticism of risk assessment. Either through a health-care system that they experience as racially discriminatory or governmental bodies that deny accountability, the residents I interviewed understand that the institutions that are now trying to document these problems through risk assessment science are the very same institutions that they feel are responsible for the problems in the first place. This is especially true around the topic of breast cancer, where African American women have increasingly lower rates of survival than any other racial or ethnic group (Walker et al. 1995; Wojcik et al. 1998). The residents I spoke with attribute this to racial discrimination that they perceive as endemic to the US healthcare system, and which has given people of colour insufficient access to services, fewer treatment options and inadequate care.

There are different ways that these informants question the 'expert' status of the health researchers and thereby assert their own claims to authenticity. One way it is expressed is within the context of the larger healthcare system, which informants feel has failed people of colour in the past, either through discriminatory practices, or through an ignorance about the needs of people of colour. As one informant said:

> The way healthcare has treated African-Americans, the quick, down dirty service, has just been totally deplorable. That's why we come in on an acute basis because we have been treated less than human. Like the doctor knows everything. No, they don't know everything. They don't understand the environmental impacts that we as African Americans and people of colour have to deal with.

Portraying the expert doctor as ignorant about the community frames him as *less* knowledgeable, having less expertise about the community, and in fact potentially posing a harm to the community members. The doctors' authenticity is called into question as a result.

Racial discrimination is also expressed in terms of the healthcare system's determination of what screening guidelines should be, and who is considered 'at risk' for certain diseases. The case of breast cancer rates in BVHP, where it is younger women that are contracting the disease, is an example of how the activists feel that their health is neglected and ignored through racial prejudices, for standard screening guidelines do not recommend mammograms for younger women. An informant explains the issue:

> The [American] Medical Association says [a minimum] age limit of fifty for breast cancer. These are the women we should screen. I've

met women as young as eighteen, nineteen years old with breast cancer. And if you don't fall within that category, you're without healthcare. So, what are we going to do when we start seeing these women at 20, 30, 40 years old? Where is the outlet for them? It's not there ... So if you don't fit perfectly in one little category, there's no room for those that slip between ... We're always excluded.

The sense of betrayal that the informants express is also placed in the context of past research that has been done, both in this community in particular and in other communities of colour more generally, in which research subjects were exploited for the benefit of the researchers, without benefit to the community. The governmental and healthcare institutions that the residents are supposed to entrust with their health have only served to disappoint and disillusion. These studies, often referred to by informants as 'Tuskegee research', have done more harm than good. Reference to the infamous Tuskegee Syphilis Experiments by the US government that took place for a large part of the twentieth century on African-American men (cf. Jones 1993) is used as an effective rhetorical and symbolic gesture and discursive device, which points out the institutional and structural history of exploitation of African-Americans in the US in the name of 'science'. This claims-making activity on the part of the activists speaks to the illegitimacy of scientific 'experts' as credible authorities within African-American communities. They may not be trustworthy to look after the best interests of those affected by environmental hazards and environmental racism.

While institutional actors were once welcomed into the community under the pretence that their intent was to improve the health of the community, the residents found that not only did the researchers exploit the residents through a scientific process that objectified them, but the research was never applied such that the community benefited from the study's results. A community activist explains the problem:

Traditionally scientists do their research and then give them a book that says 'this bunch of people ...' and then you split. Well, it can' be like that, not if you're gonna have a real effect on the popula tion and changes. And to be able to get beyond the scepticism, and historically the scepticism that African-Americans have of govern ment. How? Because it's never worked for their benefit. Tuskege and other studies that have been done. They're given very little of it ... Because what the outcome of that is that you're killing us. The people in these massive numbers in a slow way. And genocide is genocide no matter how its formulated ... You're killing us slowly, but you're still killing us.

In other words, when research is conducted in these communities, where the health effects are documented the way they often are in epidemiologic studies, the community is left in the same state as when the researcher found it, and the participants are not provided with any services or solutions: the research is conducted under false pretences. The betrayal, therefore, is the *inaction* of the institutions that are held responsible for helping improve the health and welfare of the community, and has serious and long-lasting effects on the communities 'studied'. The activists are also pointing to a structural pattern of exploitation that science consistently and institutionally repeats, whereby certain groups have research conducted on them such that other groups can benefit. As a result of their disillusionment, the BVHP community members feel they have rational reasons to distrust outside institutions that come into Bayview Hunters Point to conduct research. While institutional actors' claim that their motivations are to improve the health and welfare of the community, the community activists argue that the institutional actors' claims of credibility rather reap financial and professional benefits, often at the expense of the community affected. As the excerpt below illustrates, outside researchers come to Bayview Hunters Point to study the community and the monies that might go to helping the community instead only pay the researcher for conducting the research:

But what I do see as a big problem is that you find major institutions such as UCSF, Stanford, come in when we're at the heat of the moment, and want to come in with these prescribed prescriptions about what 'you black people need to have done'. We endorse people that want to collaborate and to work with us. But you can't give us a prescription of what we need. Saying this, I have to look at big institutions and anybody else that gets funding in the name of African-American people, but don't necessarily have the representation of those African American people. They basically extort. That's the bottom line. I have a big concern with that. And this is something that has been historical. If the health care system were intact, or doing so well ... then why are we having high rates of asthma, breast cancer? So obviously you've failed. Let's admit it. You have failed.

These institutional failings represent a larger problem for the activists in terms of how researchers interact with communities of colour. There is the perception, based on previous interactions, as seen above, that these institutional actors do not understand or want to understand the communities that they come in to study. As the same informant said later,

> A bunch of white boys sitting up on the throne, making decisions about something about my community. And not one of them lives in my community. So how dare you? That's a direct insult to me. You cannot sit here and diagnose my community living up in the ivory tower. You don't live here so how can you diagnose something going on?

Reconstruction of Risk Assessment Science

Identity politics, therefore, comes to play an important role in negotiations and debates for ownership. Like symbolic references to 'Tuskegee studies', discursive debates over the politics of representation play a crucial role for activists involved in this struggle over who they want to conduct research in their community. The racial dynamics are central. The community activists involved in this arena are all African-American. The institutional representatives are all white. For the activists I interviewed, the race of the researcher matters.[2] When asked if the community members could have it 'their way', if they would prefer an African American epidemiologist, each said that that would be important for the community. The symbolic meanings attached to 'blackness' is seen through the following statement by one informant:

> [The epidemiologist shouldn't be] just African-American. Now please understand me, because you got some people that can talk the talk but can't walk the walk. I'm talking about an African-American who knows he's African-American, as in black. And not one of these African-Americans that feel like now that I got a PhD or MD behind my name I'm moving near the white folks. Those are misdirected African-Americans ... Just because they're black

doesn't mean they're black [laughs]. Because I have seen African-American epidemiologists write studies. If I didn't know that the person was black, I would have sworn they were white.

For the community residents, racial identity and the commitments of the researcher has everything to do with the research that gets conducted. In what has been elsewhere called 'identity science' (Figert 1996) lies the notion that, concomitant with identity, whether it be racial, gendered or ethnic, are differences in practices, understandings and worldviews that affect the science that is produced. Although 'identity science' is often used as an insult by positivist scientists to those who 'let their identity get in the way' of objective research, in this case, I use the term to express the activists' critique of scientific research such that 'identities' are always present in research and research findings. In the activists' construction of identity science, colour is not enough; as the informant expresses, a racial politics is also implicated: a politics that affects the very core of the scientific endeavour. It is based on this claim that the community members negotiate their own involvement in the social arena and for control of defining environmental risk, and its causal explanations for high breast cancer rates, in Bayview. Through implying that the research that gets conducted by white researchers is biased by nature of their racial identity, the community activists are in fact making a claim that this bias creates a false objectivity of the risk assessment process. Furthermore, a researcher who identifies himself as black would conduct his or her research differently.

The 'bias' that is to them part of risk assessment within governmental and scientific institutions can only be 'undone' through community involvement in the risk assessment process. In order to achieve 'true objectivity', the partial knowledge that the risk assessors possess must be integrated with the community's knowledge, and from this union, 'objective' risk assessment can be achieved. This strategy of the community members I spoke with, to bring the community's knowledge to risk assessment, must be understood in light of the debates over the validity of the knowledge of this 'lay' public. In the early stages of the Task Force, when community activists first questioned the Department of Public Health's health assessment techniques and their findings, the Department of Public Health representatives countered the attack with a questioning of these non-experts' ability to understand this research and their ability to be 'objective' because of their emotional involvement with the issue of environmental risk. It is thus possible to read the community's critique of the 'biased' nature of 'expert' risk assessment as a further symbolic framing that points out the ways that risk assessment was not 'value-free' even before community involvement in the process. Furthermore, they claim, that it is only *through* community involvement that the science can yield valid and trustworthy results; their involvement can balance the scales in some ways. This is how an informant responded when I asked him about the biggest challenges he has faced within the Task Force:

> Some of the phenomena I've gone through before and I understand the reluctance of institutions to want to change and how it's almost a parasitical relationship ... by the Health Department in terms of them not using us to really gain from this partnering ... to truly have it integrated overall for the health of the community. That's the real problem I find – political ... It's one thing to understand science, then the politics of science. It gets in the god-damned way of doing science!

It is the 'politics of science' that has tainted the risk assessment process. The activists argue that the only way the politics can be balanced out is through community involvement at every level of the scientific process. The framing of the situation such that politics has infiltrated the sacred realm of scientific knowledge is an effective one for the community residents who are trying to authenticate the knowledge of the situation that only they, as community members, possess. Although there might be a way, in these activists' understanding of science, to conduct research 'objectively', they understand that science without politics is nearly impossible. This is why they feel that their involvement is necessary every step of the way. The authenticity of their knowledge of and their commitments to the community shapes the discourse and claims-making for their reconstruction of risk science through the importance of 'community-based research'.

Community-based Research

While 'community-based research' is a commonly used concept in public health research, what these Task Force members conceive of as 'community-based research' has far greater implications for the practice of science than that which is usually referred to as a 'community-based study'. The community members' determination to define the risk research in relation to breast cancer on their own terms is central to their claims-making activities. Above all, the activists' efforts to ensure 'inclusivity' of members of the BVHP community at every level of the research process was the primary work undertaken during my time with the Task Force. The activists' constructions and definitions of community-based research not only involve using the local community as the unit of analysis, but also means direct community involvement and input at every level of the research process.

One aspect of this construction of community-based research is that it must involve 'real-world studies'. In the community activists' experience, risk assessment in their community has meant that statistics are run on a computer in a laboratory in a university, and that the findings do not in any way represent the 'real-life' situation that the community finds itself in. Therefore, risk assessment research must be transformed to conduct tests that can tell them about their everyday conditions. Not only do the statistical tests and modelling procedures conducted not take place on the actual human bodies affected by the environment, but even when the variables are input, they do not attempt to reflect the everyday conditions of the community's members. Therefore, risk assessment must be reconstructed to attend to the issues of greatest concern to the community and to the 'real-life' conditions of residents.

As a community participant said, one of those 'real-life' conditions is the daily exposure to multiple chemicals at low levels. However, the relative risk statistics are traditionally given for a 'threshold' level of a single chemical.

> When we have a study, doctors can't even figure out what test to run on high-dose chemical exposure, not [even] low-dose multiple chemical exposure. In other words, the standards that we're using, measuring, environmental studies are not based on reality. They are based on laboratory need and economics. Therefore they are not an appropriate instrument to use to study this phenomenon we're addressing. That's part of our argument that therefore using a different approach in studying this community still needs to be resolved in the process.

The issue of uncovering a way to measure 'real life' conditions is a conundrum for cancer epidemiology in particular. Risk assessment has yet to develop adequate techniques to consider the possible links between breast cancer and the environment. In part this is due to the latency between exposures and outcomes that accompanies cancer risks, the unknown effects of human exposure to multiple chemicals, and the number of other complex variations that cannot be accounted for through risk assessment procedures. For the activists, however, the overriding reason why risk assessment science is inadequate is that its ideological and epistemological underpinnings do not allow for the possibility of including these types of risks in their equations. The unique complexity of breast cancer, with its myriad of unknowns, lies in stark contrast to the foundations of risk assessment science, which depends on isolated and discrete variables.

Furthermore, there is a way in which *environmental* risks are particularly unsuited for inclusion into risk assessment procedures which are more straightforward including quantitative, clearly demarcated variables such as age, number of children, age at first menses, etc. The uncertain and ubiquitous presence of environmental toxins cannot be reduced or quantified for inclusion in risk assessment procedures. Therefore, environmental factors for breast cancer are most often left out of the equation. What happens as a result is that the environment is eliminated as a risk factor *de facto*, because the rates, through statistical analyses, can be accounted for by the other 'known' risk factors (e.g., age, childbirth patterns, etc.). This process of elimination rules out the environment as a contributing factor, without ever having studied its possible effects. An informant speaks to this very issue:

> We have cases of women in their late twenties . . .that have cancer. One woman had seven children, okay, and she has breast cancer. Now is this a pattern? No one has done a real study, you see . . .to acknowledge the fact the environment *may* play a role in the problems here.

A related critique is that relative risk figures are traditionally based on an 'average' person, who is usually a white male. The community activists want an acknowledgement of the potential differences in risk figures for those that deviate from this 'norm'. For the activists, it is important that community-based research uses scientific standards that reflect real-world conditions, not simply a repetition of that which is considered 'traditional' research.

> This is what you're teaching in school. I'm not looking for what they taught you in school. We're looking at something totally different. Not from fifty-year-old white males' data. We're looking

for something totally unique. And the EPA [Environmental Protection Agency] standards are like that. So how you gonna compare me to a white male? First of all, you kicked us out.

Or, as another informant phrased it,

This is a multicultural society. What are the variables in it as we study different ethnic populations? California will be 51 per cent people of colour by the year 2000. How do you address that? One still finds they're still only looking at it from fifty-year-old white males' perspective. That's no good. And so with input from different communities on the research committee, on the Task Force, then we can maybe try to impact.

The breast cancer rates in BVHP present a particular example of how the community's experiences with disease demographics run counter to the statistics for the 'average' person. The statistically 'average' woman with breast cancer is white, middle-class and post-menopausal. In contrast, the 'average' woman with breast cancer in BVHP is black, poor and pre-menopausal. The activists see this contradiction not only as evidence of environmental links to breast cancer in BVHP, but also as evidence of the fact that risk assessment does not, and cannot, acknowledge the different risk factors that might exist for other types of women.

Another question for the activists is how 'risk' is statistically determined. In addition to critiques of scientific objectivity, these activists also question the foundations of scientific validity. One informant expresses this in terms of the breast cancer rates in BVHP:

I'm [seeing] elevated rates! 'Well, it's not statistically significant where it's two powers . . .' Elevated period. If it's anything over one it's elevated. What's happening? You know? How many got to die, damn it? The body count isn't high enough?

This sentiment lies at the heart of many environmental justice claims that the standards of scientific validity have nothing whatsoever to do with caring for human lives. The morbid portrayal of scientists 'counting' human bodies speaks symbolically to this point and to the previous discussion about the researchers' underlying motives in studying communities 'at risk'.

Perhaps most important to the community activists I interviewed is the concept that there should be community involvement and consent at every level of research, and moreover that community members should lead the research teams whenever possible. The activists understand that changing the institutional structures and the deeply embedded ideas about how scientific research should be conducted is an uphill battle, with profound resistance from the 'experts' on the Task Force. In the following excerpts, two informants describe resistance from the health researchers and epidemiologists on the Task Force, yet simultaneously envisage changes:

> We have to have every party at the table. Those who are affected as well as those who are studying the phenomenon, jointly studying together. Not this hierarchy of I'm God and I'm talking to you down below. You need a multiple-disciplinary approach, and in the process of doing it you want to improve health in the situation and you teach the residents.

> I see a resolution, once the great white hope realize it's not just them involved. It's the community that has the solutions to most of the problems. And them being true players in remedying some of those problems. You think you're gonna come into my community to do outreach over here? [They] bring a whole bunch of white people to do outreach. Why couldn't you hire people from my own community to do outreach on themselves? ...I'm saying that crap is over with. People are sick of it. It's not gonna happen anymore.

For these activists, community resident involvement at the ground-level of any scientific research endeavour is the only way to improve both the practices of scientific research in their community as well as their health. The partnership that they envisage between governmental authorities and community residents is dependent on an ideological and epistemological shift for the production of risk knowledge, such that the determination of authoritative knowledge is not based merely on 'scientific' claims. Rather they see change emerging from a dialogic process between 'experts' and the community, whereby both 'parties' realize that the residents' authentic status as 'community members' is a valuable, credible and knowledgeable location for the understanding of environmental risk in BVHP.

Conclusion

While contestation over the practice of scientific research is only one of many activist endeavours in the Bayview Hunters Point community and within the Task Force, it stands out as one of the primary areas where these community residents are having an impact on the traditional practices of local government agencies and politics. The community activists I spoke with well understand that science has consequences. However, the bases on which they feel that authoritative scientific claims should be made delineate a very different way of conducting community-based research and of generating scientific knowledge from the traditional methodological paradigm. The credibility struggles that the activists in Bayview Hunters Point engage in with local risk experts highlight the nature of the residents' resistance to traditional scientific approaches and practices, and simultaneously reconstruct the risk assessment process to account for the activists' own conceptions of credibility, authority and authenticity. Their claims to authenticity and to credible 'expertise' in their own right are founded on their first-hand knowledge and experiences as members of the local community; on their racial identities and political commitments to improving the health in the community; and on a critique of science and scientific and healthcare institutions as untrustworthy, racially discriminatory and inadequate. Based on documentation of elevated rates of breast cancer and the overwhelming presence of toxic hazards in their community, the Bayview Hunters Point residents engage with the production of scientific knowledge in order to (re)construct risk assessment to account for this reality. The activists are arguing that science can have consequences other than negative ones, wherein inadequate and incomplete risk information becomes reified and concretized as the 'truth' through ideas about the 'average' breast cancer patient and who is deemed at risk and who is not. Rather, if conducted with community involvement and with appropriate attention paid to the local community's unique (class, racial, social, cultural and environmental) positioning, the production of risk knowledge can bring money and resources to a community that desperately needs them and a means and methods of improving the health conditions for the community's residents.

Notes

1   The Superfund Program was established in the United States in 1980 by the

Comprehensive, Response, Compensation, and Liability Act (CERCLA) to create priority lists and to provide funds for clean-up of the worst hazardous waste sites in the US. As of December 1998, there were 1,192 Superfund sites on the Final National Priority List (NPL), a list of the most serious sites identified for possible long-term remedial response. Sixty-six sites, as of December 1998, are currently proposed to be added to the NPL. (http://www.epa.gov/oerrpage/superfnd/web/sites/)

2 At this point, the reader may be wondering about my own race and identity, as a researcher in BVHP, and perhaps more pointedly how I attained entrée into the fieldsite given the community's distrust of researchers in general. As a white researcher from UCSF, an academic and medical institution that the activists had some previous (negative) interactions with, I knew that access might be difficult. I used a couple of different strategies to earn the trust of the residents. First and foremost was the fact that I approached the Task Force members who were community residents to ask their permission to work with them on the Task Force. Because of my connections to UCSF, I could have approached the public health 'experts' on the Task Force to get access to Task Force members and activities. However, in the residents' eyes, this would have immediately aligned me with the Department of Public Health's representatives, as opposed to the residents. Therefore, in my attempts to understand the community's feelings and attitudes about environmental links to breast cancer, I made a conscious decision to 'align' myself with the residents. But earning their trust was not automatic. In some ways I spent the first month or two in the field 'proving' myself to the residents. The trust that developed between us arose as a result of the community activists' feelings that they and I came from similar ideological, political and epistemological standpoints, particularly around the issue of environmental justice. In fact, it was after I revealed to them that I too was critical of risk assessment science that they more readily welcomed me into their meetings and ongoing activities. The second strategy I employed was to assume that the residents were the most knowledgeable about issues of environmental risk in their neighbourhood, and that I was there to learn from them about their community and about their experiences. Third, I allowed the activists to employ me as a messenger, whereby I was expected to carry their message and sentiments about scientific research back to my institution and the researchers there. Perhaps more broadly, they also saw me as a way to get their message out to an even broader audience, for there was an understanding that I would be writing and publishing my findings from my work with the Task Force.

References

Abraham, J. and J. Sheppard. 'Democracy, Technocracy and the Secret State of Medicine's Control: Expert and Nonexpert Perspectives'. *Science, Technology, and Human Values* 22 (1997) pp. 139–67.

Aragon, T. and K. Grumbach. *Community Health Profile* (San Francisco: The Bayview Health and Environmental Assessment Task Force 1997).

Bayview Hunters Point Health and Environmental Task Force. *Community*

Toxics Profile (San Francisco: The Bayview Hunters Point Health and Environmental Assessment Task Force 1996).

Beck, U. *Risk Society: Towards a New Modernity* (London, Sage 1992).

Bullard, R.D. 'Solid Waste Sites and the Black Houston Community'. *Sociological Inquiry* 53 (1983) pp. 273–88.

Clarke, L. and J. Short, Jr. 'Social Organization and Risk: Some Current Controversies'. *Annual Review of Sociology* 19 (1993) pp. 375–99.

Commission for Racial Justice. *Toxic Wastes and Race in the United States: A National Report on the Racial and Socio-Economic Characteristics of Communities With Hazardous Waste Sites* (New York: Commission for Racial Justice 1987).

Douglas, M. *Risk and Blame: Essays in Cultural Theory* (New York: Routledge 1992).

Environmental Law and Justice Clinic. *Bayview-Hunter's Point Community Environmental Guide* (San Francisco: Southeast Alliance for Environmental Justice 1998).

Epstein, S. *Impure Science: AIDS, Activism, and the Politics of Knowledge* (Berkeley, University of California Press 1996).

Figert, A.E. *Women and the Ownership of PMS: The Structuring of a Psychiatric Disorder* (New York: Aldine de Gruyter 1996).

Freudenburg, W.R. 'Risk and Recreancy: Weber, the Division of Labor, and the Rationality of Risk Perceptions'. *Social Forces* 71 (1993) pp. 909–32.

Glazer, B. and A. Strauss. *The Discovery of Grounded Theory* (Chicago: Aldine 1967).

Hammersley, M. and P. Atkinson. *Ethnography: Principles in Practice* (London: Routledge 1966).

Jacobs, J. and L. Dopkeen. 'Risking the Qualitative Study of Risk'. *Qualitative Sociology* 13 (1990) pp. 169–81.

Johnson, C. 'Bayview-Hunters Point Sick of Industrial Fumes'. *San Francisco Chronicle* (1995).

Jones, J.H. *Bad Blood: The Tuskegee Syphilis Experiment* (New York: The Free Press 1993).

Lambert, H. and H. Rose. 'Disembodied Knowledge? Making Sense of Medical Science'. A. Irwin and B. Wynne, eds. *Misunderstanding Science? The Public Reconstruction of Science and Technology* (Cambridge: Cambridge University Press, 1996).

McKechnie, R. 'Insiders and Outsiders: Identifying Experts on Home Ground'. A. Irwin and B. Wynne, eds. *Misunderstanding Science? The Public Reconstruction of Science and Technology* (Cambridge: Cambridge University Press, 1996).

Perhac, R.M., Jr. 'Comparative Risk Assessment: Where Does the Public Fit In?' *Science, Technology, and Human Values* 23 (1998) pp. 221–41.

Prior, L. 'Chance and Modernity: Accidents as a Public Health Problem'. R. Bunton, S. Nettleton and R. Burrows, eds. *The Sociology of Health Promotion* (London: Routledge 1995).

Robinson, J.C. 'Racial Inequality and the Probability of Occupation-Related Injury or Illness'. *Milbank Memorial Fund Quarterly: Health and Society* 62 (1984) pp. 567–90.

San Francisco Chronicle Staff. 'S.F. Cancer Study Finds Baffling Rates in Bayview'. *San Francisco Chronicle* (1995).

Shrader-Frechette, K.S. *Risk and Rationality* (Berkeley: University of California Press, 1991).

Silbergeld, E.K. 'Risk Assessment and Risk Management: An Uneasy Divorce'. D.G. Mayo and R.D. Hollander, eds. *Acceptable Evidence: Science and Values in Risk Management* (New York: Oxford University Press 1991).

Spradley, J.P. *Participant Observation* (New York: Harcourt Brace Jovanovich College Publishers 1980).

Strauss, A. and J. Corbin. *Basics of Qualitative Research: Grounded Theory Procedures and Techniques* (Newbury Park: Sage Publications, Inc., 1990).

Vaughan, E. and B. Nordenstam. 'The Perception of Environmental Risks among Ethnically Diverse Groups'. *Journal of Cross-Cultural Psychology* 2 (1991) pp. 29–60.

Walker, B., L.W. Figgs. and S.H. Zahm. 'Differences in Cancer Incidence, Mortality, and Survival Between African Americans and Whites'. *Environmental Health Perspectives* 103 (1995) pp. 275–81.

Wojcik, B., M.K. Spinks and S.A. Optenberg. 'Breast Carcinoma Survival Analysis for African American and White Women in an Equal-Access Health Care System, *Cancer* 82 (1998) pp. 1310–18.

Wynne, B. 'Misunderstood Misunderstandings: Social Identities and Public Uptake of Science'. A. Irwin and B. Wynne, eds. *Misunderstanding Science? The Public Reconstruction of Science and Technology* (Cambridge: Cambridge University Press, 1996).

Index

Acker, K., 9, 54–5, 108, 113, 116, 120
activism, 15, 63–93, 92n, 181, 185,
    189, 199
    see also feminism; women's health
    movement
African American, 186, 187, 193
    see also black women; racism;
    women of colour
Ahmed, S., 108, 117, 120, 123
AIDS, 65
    activism, inspiration of, 75, 76, 79
    quilt, 73
alternative medicine, 5, 54, 106, 116,
    119
Althusser, L., 2, 88
American Cancer Society, 83, 86
anger, 45, 53, 65–6, 79, 84, 88
Anglin, M.K., 65, 66–7, 67
Anzaldua, G., 124
autobiography, 54, 99, 106, 99, 119,
    122
    and feminism (*q.v.*), 102, 105
    traditional masculine genre of,
    98, 101, 102, 104, 112

Bartky, S.L., 157, 164–5, 169, 174,
    175, 176
Batt, S., 64, 100, 103, 108, 110
Bayview Hunters Point (San
    Francisco), 85, 181–201 *passim*,
    182, 185, 186
beauty, 43, 89–90, 122
    challenges to, 78
    see also body – idealized, breasts;
    fashion
Beck, U., 183
Becker, H., 17, 24
    see also credibility
Benstock, S., 112, 118, 119, 121, 122
biomedicine, 7, 16, 18, 29, 30, 35, 90
    and Race for the Cure (*q.v.*), 87
    see also medicine; power; science

biopsy, 22, 24, 25
black women, 52
    see also African Americans;
    racism; women of colour
blame, *see* responsibility
body, 20, 38, 42, 118
    alienation from, 105, 122
    altered, 58, 87, 89, 117, 122, 165;
    and *see* mastectomy;
    mutilation; reconstruction
    artistic presentation of, 53, 55
    Cixous on, 105
    corporeal styles, 77–8, 88–9
    dangerous, 8, 145, 160–9
    feminine, *see* femininity
    gendered, 164, 175; and *see*
    femininity, gender
    idealized, 78, 166
    identity and (*q.v.*), 164
    incomplete, 172
    integrity of, 169, 174
    male gaze and (*q.v.*), 39, 164, 165
    management of, *see* disciplinary
    practices
    'other' than self, 156, 173
    out of control, 162, 163
    parts, 156, 157
    social construction of, 157
Brady, J., 86, 93n
Braidotti, R., 117, 123
breasts, 37, 55, 164, 170, 175
    femininity (*q.v.*) and, 39, 165–6,
    174
    idealization of, 38, 43, 169
    identity (*q.v.*) and, 52, 174
    maternalized, 40
    normalization of, 8, 175; and *see*
    reconstruction
    relation to self, 115–16, 156
    sexualization of, 37, 39
    see also mastectomy; sexuality
breast cancer, 40, 51, 106, 115, 161

breast cancer – *continued*
   statistics, 1, 15, 41, 80, 85, 93n,
      143, 153, 182, 187, 199
   and young women, 41
   see also heredity; narratives
Breast Cancer Awareness Month, 1,
      15, 70, 74, 82–3
   see also Race for the Cure; Toxic
      Tour of the Cancer Industry
breast cancer movement, 63–4, 65,
      66, 90, 146
   see also self-help groups; social
      movements
breast cancer organizations, 63, 64,
      66
   see also Komen Foundation
Breast Cancer Prevention Trial, *see*
      tamoxifen
breast self-examination, 6, 21, 30–1,
      41, 74
   see also screening
Brinker, Nancy, 69, 74
   see also Komen Foundation
Brodski and Schenk, 104, 105
Brohn, P., 106, 109, 116
Butler, J., 77–8, 104, 124
Butler, S. and Rosenblum, B., 101,
      102, 106, 108, 110, 111, 113,
      114

cancer, 84, 112
   meanings and understandings of,
      1, 28, 38–9, 104, 156
   stories of, 109
cancer industry, 5–6, 15, 65, 71, 82
   constituents of, 83, 86
   see also Toxic Tour of the Cancer
      Industry, 83–7
carcinogens, 6, 32, 82, 89, 146, 147,
      148, 197–8
   see also causation; risk
Carson, R., 6
Cartwright, L., 42, 43, 44, 102, 108
causation, 15, 82, 137,
   environmental, 6, 147–8, 181
   questions of, 19, 74, 108
   see also carcinogens; oestrogen
choice, 5
   and prophylactic mastectomy

(*q.v.*), 47–8
   see also decision-making
Cixous, H., 101, 105
Cohan, S. and Shires, L.M., 111, 114
Colbourn, C., 113
Cole, J., 99, 100, 101, 106, 108, 110,
      111, 113, 116, 121
'coming out', 72, 120, 123
   see also identity; stories
community, 72–3, 77, 90, 181, 187,
      200
   at risk, 182, 184
   see also research
consciousness raising, 98, 99, 100,
      102, 104, 125n
   see also identity; self – new sense
      of
consent, informed
   to research, 200
   to treatment, 65–6
   see also decision-making
control, 5, 29, 110, 162, 163
   cancer as out of control, 38–9,
      104, 105, 108, 109
   medical, 146; and *see*
      biomedicine
credibility
   hierarchy of, 24
   struggles, 17, 184–5, 189–90
Culler, J., 108
culture, 18–19, 68, 122
   cultures of action, 63, 65, 87, 88
   and social movements, 67–9
cure, 32–3
   see also Race for the Cure

Dale, E., 113, 114, 115, 121
danger, 131, 161, 166
   in environment (*q.v.*), 182
   Foucault (*q.v.*) on, 160
dangerous body parts, 160, 162, 168,
      175
Datan, N., 4
Davis, D.L. and Bradlow, L., 148
death, 33–4, 38, 47, 55, 58, 87
   images of, 79, 85, 89
   writing against, 101
decision-making
   about prophylactic surgery (*q.v.*),

47, 48, 162, 166, 168
about risk management (*q.v.*),
132, 140, 141, 142, 143
about treatment, 51, 54
detection, 21, 23, 25, 26, 82, 113, 114
accidental, 27, 28
early, 30, 65, 73–4, 77, 86, 144,
168
diagnosis, 22, 25, 39, 74, 90, 114
diaries, 98, 99, 113, 121
disciplinary practices, 164, 176
see also femininity
disease, 114, 136, 137, 145
meanings and understandings of,
21, 106, 108
social construction of, 20
stories (*q.v.*) of, 109
disfigurement, 43, 85, 122
see also mastectomy; mutilation
Duncker, P., 106, 125 ref.

embodiment, 69, 78, 88, 99, 117,
174, 175
gendered (*q.v.*), 175–6
of knowledge (*q.v.*), 21–2
of self (*q.v.*), 174
empowerment, 7–8, 162, 164
environment, 80, 137
and risk (*q.v.*), 147, 148, 150, 155
environmental hazards, 83, 85, 86,
137, 181, 186, 192
see also causation; risk
environmental justice, 65, 81, 83, 87,
90, 188, 199
environmental organizations, 5, 81,
181, 182, 197
environmental racism, 65, 84, 87,
182, 186, 187, 192
epidemiology, *see* breast cancer;
statistics
Epstein, S., 6, 184, 185,
ethnicity, 140
see also African Americans; black
women; racism; women of
colour
experience, women's lived, 2, 16, 29,
30, 32, 34
specificity of, 51, 100, 103, and
see social positioning

shared, 72, 99, 100, 102, 103
experts, 23, 25, 29, 109, 181, 185,
189, 190, 192, 200, 201

family, obligations to, 163, 168
history of breast cancer, *see*
heredity
fashion, 42, 55, 71
fear, 37, 47, 103, 106, 131, 137, 162,
164
Felman, S., 121
femininity, 8, 9, 37, 45, 164
and the body (*q.v.*), 8, 39, 160,
175
and breasts (*q.v.*), 165, 174
challenges to, 55, 58, 78, 79, 165,
174
compromised, 8, 168–9, 170, 173
hetero-, 65, 78, 89
'natural', 164, 165, 167
norms of, 9, 44, 65, 66, 70, 165,
166, 175
violation of, 43, 44
see also disciplinary practices
feminism, 2, 4, 8, 20, 29, 65, 75,
110
and activism (*q.v.*), 65–7, 78, 81,
84
Figert, A.E., 195
Flax, J., 102
Foucault, M.
dangerous bodies (*q.v.*), 160
medical gaze (*q.v.*), 17, 20
subjugated knowledges (*q.v.*), 24,
35n, 68, 90, 117
Friedman, S.S., 102, 110, 119
Fugh-Bergman, A., 144, 146
Fuss, D., 2, 118, 119

gaze
male, 40, 170; and *see* body;
breasts
medical, 9n, 17, 20–3
gender
identity, 43, 52, 59, 174, 175–6,
178–9n; challenges to, 54, 66;
'natural', 160, 164–5 as
institution, 66
social construction of, 164

genes, 47, 48, 49,
　BRCA1&2, 7, 153
　genetic mutation, 45, 153, 154,
　　161
　see also heredity; risk
Giddens, A., 8, 164, 174
Gifford, S., 144
Goel, V., 141–2
grounded theory, 17, 189
groups, *see* breast cancer
　organizations; self-help groups

hair loss, 52, 56, 57, 58, 122
　and lesbian/queer aesthetic, 78
health
　issues, 37, 84, 148
　political-economy model of, *see*
　　politics of breast cancer
healthcare, 5, 8
　inequalities in, 75, 80 ,87, 191;
　　and *see* racism
heredity, 7, 45, 133, 139, 153, 157,
　158, 176
　breast cancer families, 46, 153–4,
　　158
heroism, *see* narratives – heroic
heterofemininity, 78, 89
　see also femininity
hiddenness, 39, 79
　of breast cancer, 28, 44, 53, 69,
　　113
　of effects of treatment, 44
　see also visibility
hormones, *see* oestrogen
horror, 38, 44–5, 46, 51, 58
HRT, 141,148
　see also oestrogen
Hubbard, R., 148–9

iatrogenesis
　of mammography (*q.v.*), 32, 154
　of risk management (*q.v.*), 155
　of treatment, 56
identity, 104, 116, 117, 118, 122,
　164
　and the feminine body, 165, 168
　politics, 194
　racial, 185, 194–5, 201
　'at risk' (*q.v.*), 155

as survivor (*q.v.*), 64, 66, 72, 74, 89
as victim (*q.v.*), 81, 86, 89
as warrior, 124
as woman living with breast
　cancer, 37, 87, 88, 105, 118,
　123, 124
see also body; femininity; self
ideology, 1–2, 4, 88, 131, 135, 141,
　149
　and culture, 67
　of personal responsibility (*q.v.*),
　　136–7, 143, 145
　of social responsibility (*q.v.*), 137,
　　147, 148–9
　of technology (*see also* science),
　　88, 135, 141, 149
　see also femininity; values
illness, 37, 58, 102, 120
images, *see* breasts; death;
　femininity; mastectomy
implants, 85, 155, 167
　see also reconstruction; risk
isolation, 102, 104
　see also experience, women's lived

Joolz, 99
Julien, J., 105, 109, 112, 115, 121

Kavanagh, A.M. and Broom, D.H.,
　155–6, 163, 174
Kelly, M.P. and Field, D., 117, 121
Kent, J., 169
Klausner, M.D., 139, 144
knowledge, 16, 22, 29, 99, 100, 163,
　184
　biomedical, 21, 23, 25, 32; and *see*
　　biomedicine
　embodied, 21, 23, 25, 26, 30; and
　　see biomedicine
　expert (*q.v.*), 23, 195, 200
　legitimacy of, 18, 23, 24, 29, 34,
　　94
　multiplicity of, 15, 21, 23
　and power (*q.v.*), 24, 195
　production of, 182, 184, 185, 189,
　　200
　scientific, 18, 182, 184; and *see*
　　science
　social construction of, 18

subjugated, 23–8, 90
women's, 16, 21, 24, 28, 29, 30
see also experience women's,
lived; uncertainty
Komen Foundation, 69–70, 73, 77,
82–3, 92–3n
see also Brinker, Nancy
Kristeva, J., 118

Lacan, J. 119, 121
lesbian women, 9, 52, 75
and queer, 78
lifestyle, 8, 19, 86, 136, 141, 146, 155
see also risk
Lock, M., 145
Lorber, J., 66
Lorde, A., 8, 52, 100–1, 103, 104, 106,
110, 113, 117, 118, 121, 122–3,
124
loss, 44, 50
of breast, 44, 47, 156, 165–6, 169,
171–2; and *see* mastectomy
of self (*q.v.*), 120, 122
Love, Dr. S., 6–7, 103
lumps, 21, 22–3, 25, 26, 113, 116
Lynch, D. and Richards, E., 103, 106,
109, 110, 114, 116, 121–2

mammography, 24, 30–2, 70, 74
failures of, 26, 93
images of, 41
mass programmes, 6–7
randomness of, 27
risks of, 41
and young women, 61n, 154, 191
see also screening
Margolese, R., 141
Martin, E., 156–7, 163, 174
mastectomy, 38, 43, 156
and identity (*q.v.*), 157, 165
images of, 43–5, 53, 55, 63, 79, 85
prophylactic, *see* prophylaxis
see also breasts; femininity; loss;
media; mutilation; prosthesis;
visibility
maternity, 47, 48–51, 57
see also family
Matuschka, 53, 63–4
see also mastectomy, images of

Mayer, M., 100, 101, 102, 103, 109,
110, 111, 112, 117–18, 120, 121
McTiernan, A. et al., 143
meanings, 1, 2, 100, 108
narrative construction of, 2,
106–11, 114
media representation, 32, 37–61,
59–60n
emphasis on youth, 38, 41
of risk (*q.v.*), 137
of science (*q.v.*) 140
see also images
medical gaze, *see* gaze, clinical
medical profession, 8, 105, 109, 110,
120, 191
see also 'experts'; medicine
medicine, 102, 145
dependency on, 144, 145, 150
progress in, 74, 136, 144; and *see*
modernity
see also biomedicine; knowledge;
science
menopause, 40–1
Minh–ha, Trinh T., 119
mirrors, 121–2
see also self-image
modernity,
and medical progress, 5, 6, 74, 75;
and *see* medicine; biomedicine
and risk (*q.v.*), 183, 184
Montini, T., 65–6, 67
mortality,
in 'high-risk' groups, 154
and tamoxifen (*q.v.*) 142
see also breast cancer; death;
statistics
multiculturalism, 65, 75, 79, 199
multinational industries, 71, 79, 83,
85, 136
see also Cancer Industry Tour;
causation; environment
mutilation, 43, 45, 46, 90
see also mastectomy

narratives, 98–124
anti-normative, 54, 57
cancer, 45–51
collective/shared, 101–2
forms and structures of, 111–14

narratives *continued*
  heroic, 49, 110, 111
  master, 110, 117, 124
  published, 121, 123
  purposes of, 98, 99, 100
  self-discovery, 106
  tragic, 51, 57
  see also stories; texts
normativization of women's
    experiences (*q.v.*), 52, 109, 111

objectivity, 16, 18, 19, 183, 190
  critique of, 20, 132, 195
  see also biomedicine; knowledge;
    science
oestrogen, 138, 146, 147
  manipulation of, 146, 147
  mimics, 147, 148
  role in causation (*q.v.*), 20, 147–8
  see also environment; HRT; pill
Orr, J., 20

Picardie, R., 54, 55–9
pill (contraceptive), 141, 148
  see also oestrogen
politics, 19, 54, 86, 137
  and causation (*q.v.*), 148
  of personal experience, 100
  of prevention (*q.v.*), 132, 149
  racial, 195
  of risk assessment (*q.v.*), 183, 184
power, 67, 68
  and knowledge (*q.v.*), 24, 29
  and the medical profession (*q.v.*),
    66
  and the 'relations of ruling', 29
  through writing, 119
  see also resistance
predictive testing, 154, 158
  see also genes
prevention, 84, 131, 138, 144, 150,
    162
  chemo-prevention, 135, 138–44,
    148; and *see* tamoxifen
  and early detection, 31
  and the environment (*q.v.*), 86–7,
    90, 147–8
  primary, 5, 65, 137, 147–8
  see also prophylaxis

Pritchard, K., 142
Proctor, R., 88–9, 137
prognosis, *see* cure; mortality;
    survival
prophylaxis, 8, 31, 154
  chemo-prevention, *see* tamoxifen
  surgical (*see also* mastectomy),
    45–9, 141, 154, 158, 161, 173
prosthesis, 52, 53, 71, 89
  resistance (*q.v.*) to, 78, 117
  see also mastectomy;
    reconstruction

Race for the Cure, 64, 69–75, 82, 87
racism, 140, 182, 191
  see also environmental racism;
    healthcare systems; inequalities
radiation, 32, 154, 168
  see also environment;
    mammography
RavenLight, 78–9, 89
  see also mastectomy images
reconstruction, 8, 53, 78, 118
  of breast, 59, 89, 158, 166, 170,
    171, 175; and *see* breasts,
    femininity
  of identity, 156, 169, 173; and *see*
    self, new
recurrence, 22, 28, 33,
relationships, *see* sexuality
research, 5, 17, 19, 195
  agenda, 132, 133, 145, 146, 147
  biomedical, 65, 73, 77; and *see*
    biomedicine; science
  community involvement in, 190,
    192, 194, 195, 196, 200
  exploitative, 192, 193, 194; and
    see racism
  methods: case studies, 157–60;
    grounded theory, 17, 189;
    participant observation, 64,
    92n, 93n, 188
  racism in, 140, 182, 191
  'real-world studies', 197, 198
  see also risk assessment
resistance, 57, 181, 182, 185
  Foucault on, 117
  Rowbotham on, 124
  Said on, 109

through writing, 110, 120
responsibility
  collective, 147
  for detection (*q.v.*), 31
  to family (*q.v.*), 163, 168
  of institutions, 192, 193
  personal/individual, 31, 33, 74,
    136, 143, 145, 146
  social, 137
Rich, A., 106
risk, 8, 131–50, 160, 183
  assessment, 7, 133–5, 138, 143,
    149, 145, 181–5, 189,
    197
  data, 19–20, 132, 133, 181
  embodied, 155, 166
  environmental (*q.v.*), 1, 5, 184,
    185, 186, 197–8
  factors, 139, 143, 198; and *see*
    causation
  'high-risk' women, 7–8, 139, 140,
    144, 154, 155, 158–60, 181
  individual, 71, 133, 134, 144, 153,
    155–6
  inherited, 45, 133; and *see* genes,
    heredity
  reduction, 145, 148; and *see*
    prevention
  social, 137; and see prevention
  see also decision-making;
    implants; mammography;
    tamoxifen; values
Robertson, A., 162
Rose, H., 4
Rowbotham, S., 122, 123, 124

sacrifice, 48–51, 168
  see also family
Said, E., 109
San Francisco Bay Area, 6, 9n, 64–93
  passim, 80, 87, 93n 182
science, 8, 133, 135, 184, 195
  and biomedicine (*q.v.*), 18, 65
  challenges to, 18, 185
  and credibility (*q.v.*), 189, 190
  and knowledge (*q.v.*), 133, 183,
    201
  politics of, 196
  and risk (*q.v.*), 132, 145, 183, 189

screening, 155
  for 'high risk' women (*q.v.*), 154,
    168
  see also mammography
Sedgewick, E., 43–4, 52
Segrave, E., 110, 113
self, 98, 103, 105, 111, 117, 118, 119,
    121, 173
  authentic, 118, 119, 120, 121
  core, 117, 118
  essentialist notion of, 118, 119
  fragmented, 116, 119, 121, 156
  new sense of, 100, 104, 115, 116,
    117, 120, 121
  relation to the body (*q.v.*), 118,
    156–7
  threats to, 120, 156, 165
  see also body; femininity; identity
self-help groups, 5, 34, 66, 103, 108,
    158
self-image, 48, 165
  in mirror, 121–2
sexuality, 47, 59, 169
  and breasts (*q.v.*), 52, 170–1
  challenges to norms of, 55, 78
  sexual relationships, 47, 48, 167,
    172
Shildrick, M., 105, 164
Shrader-Frechette, K.S., 133–4, 183
silence, 39, 53, 90, 106, 123
  resistance to, 72, 101, 106
Simmonds, F.N., 115, 115–6
sisterhood, 100, 103, 104
Smith, D., 2–3, 4, 5, 29–30
social construction
  of body (*q.v.*), 157
  of disease (*q.v.*), 20
  of gender (*q.v.*), 176
  of knowledge (*q.v.*), 18
social movements, 64, 67–9, 185
  see also activism; breast cancer
    movement; cultures of action
social positioning, 16, 51, 59, 81,
    102, 108, 118, 186, 199, 201
  and class, 17–18
  privileged, 67, 149
sociology, 3, 65, 91
  feminist, 2, 29
  of knowledge (*q.v.*), 29, 66

solidarity, 69, 88, 100, 123, 124
   see also activism
Solomon, A., 40
Sontag, S.,1, 38, 58, 108, 156, 161
Spence, J., 99, 103, 105, 106, 109,
   110, 111, 115, 116, 118
   with David Roberts, 107
Stacey, J., 1, 38, 43, 50, 58, 109, 110,
   118–19, 120, 156
Stanley, L., 98, 103, 114, 120, 123
statistics, *see* breast cancer; statistics
Steingraber, S., 6
stigma, 72, 86, 90
stories, 25, 91, 98–9, 101, 108, 115
   personal, 81, 98–124
   shared, 101–3, 104
   story telling, 99, 108, 111, 119
   see also experiences, women's;
      narratives; texts
subject
   asserting presence of, 2, 105
   of own life story (*q.v.*), 109, 112,
      118, 119
   positions, 117, 123
subjectivity, 92n, 98, 101, 123–4,
   172
surgery, *see* mastectomy;
   reconstruction
surveillance, 6, 8, 140, 156, 161, 168
   see also risk management;
      screening
survival, 72–3, 73, 74, 104–5, 105,
   164, 168
   see also cure
survivors, 64, 66, 74, 77
   images of, 55, 73
   and Komen Foundation (*q.v.*), 69
   and the Race for the Cure (*q.v.*), 72
   see also identity
Swidler, A., 68

tamoxifen, 82, 93, 135, 138–44,
   150n,
   action of, 138–9, 142
   BCPT (*q.v.*), 139–42
   and minority ethnic women, 140
   risk assessment, 135, 140, 141,
      143, 145
   side-effects, 139, 141

   see also prophylaxis, chemo-
      prevention; Zeneca
Taylor, V. and van Willigen, M., 65,
   66, 67
technology, *see* ideology; science
testimony, 98
   see also narrative; stories
texts, 29, 99, 101
   and identity (*q.v.*), 119
   see also narratives; stories
Toxic Links Coalition, 81-3, 93n
Toxic Tour of the Cancer Industry, 6,
   65, 81–7, 87
truth, 19, 23, 29, 99
   see also knowledge
Turner, B., 120

uncertainty
   of BSE (*q.v.*), 30
   of cancer (*q.v.*), 109, 161
   of knowledge (*q.v.*), 19, 22, 23,
      24, 27, 28, 140, 141, 142, 143
   of risk assessment (*q.v.*), 143, 144,
      176, 181, 198

values, 34, 132, 133, 134, 183
   and research (*q.v.*), 145–6
   'value-free', 184, 196; and *see*
      objectivity
Veronesi, P. et al., 142
vested interests, 15, 82, 136, 145
victims, 81, 86, 89; and *see*
   identity
visibility, 2, 72, 78, 106, 123
Voda, A.M., 40

Walder, J., 103, 113, 115
Waller, M. and Batt, S., 146
Waugh, P., 102, 110, 123
Wilber, K., 121
Wittig, M., 124
Women and Cancer Walk, 65, 75–81,
   87
women of colour, 73, 84, 186
   see also African Americans; black
      women; racism
women's health movement, 4, 17,
   65, 99, 110
women's health organizations, 75, 77

women's liberation movement, 98
   see also feminism
writing, 101, 105, 106, 110, 119

Yardley, L., 102

Yorke, L., 106
Young, I., 164, 165, 169, 172, 175

Zeneca, 1, 9n, 82, 138